Leadership questions and forms of working in the anthropososphic medical movement

Leadership questions and forms of working in the anthroposophic medical movement

Edited by Michaela Glöckler
and Rolf Heine
for the International Coordination
of Anthroposophic Medicine/IKAM

Verlag am Goetheanum

Translated by Christian von Arnim

www.vamg.ch

Cover-Design: Wolfram Schildt, Berlin, by using a picture of Gertrud von Heydebrand-Osthoff, Staatsarchiv Basel-Stadt, BSL 1023 1-4-14-1a

Typesetting: Höpcke, Hamburg
Printing and binding: Druckhaus Nomos, Sinzheim

ISBN 978-3-7235-1584-6

Contents

Dedicated in gratitude to:

Erika von Arnim (1918–2007)
Rita Leroi (1913–1988)
Rudolf Grosse (1905–1994)
Thomas McKeen (1953–1993)
Bernard Lievegoed (1905–1992)
Margarete Kirchner-Bockholt (1894–1973)

The healthy social life is found
When in the mirror of each human soul
The whole community finds its reflection
And when in the community
The virtue of each one is living.

Motto of social ethics,
5 November 1920*

---

* From Steiner, R.; Maryon, E.: *Briefwechsel – Briefe – Sprüche – Skizzen 1912–1924* (GA 263/1). Rudolf Steiner Verlag, Dornach 1990.

Foreword to the fourth edition

Since the publication of this book at Easter 2010, we have received a gratifying number of questions about its content as well as suggestions as to how to make it better understood. This motivated us thoroughly to revise the book for the fourth edition. "Us" means the members of the International Coordination of Anthroposophic Medicine / IKAM who are responsible for this publication.

Why do we consider it important to describe the positive intentions underlying the leadership questions and forms of working set out her? On the one hand this is a piece of living history of the anthroposophic medical movement, what we might call its "organisation chart" as it has taken shape since 1988, including internationally. On the other hand we set out our attempt to realise the modes of working for which Rudolf Steiner sowed the seeds for the anthroposophical movement at the 1923/1924 Christmas Conference.

In her foreword to the book published about the Christmas Conference, Marie Steiner wrote that all the negotiations documented in it were a path of schooling relating to the management of meetings and dealing with the problems of the Society.[1] It therefore seemed an obvious step to take up this approach also with regard to the social organisational processes in the anthroposophic medical movement. Taking this path of schooling seriously and testing the potential power of its social impact thus became our task; and it kept providing us with new inspiration.

We were therefore happy to include in this new edition the questions and perspectives which arose from numerous discussions with and letters from co-workers of the anthroposophic medical movement. They are included in the new chapter "Questions and answers about our leadership concept". We hope that this will illustrate even more clearly the extent to which an international working community, whose aim is to help and heal, requires social forms which correspond to this impulse. In this context the “Motto of social ethics” quoted above has provided a basic guideline. Because a healthy and inspiring social culture does not arise until the particular contributions of the individual co-workers in the organisations and institutions are received in such a way that these co-workers can not only give of their best but are also supported by the community in doing so. It is our concern to keep working on such a social culture.

In order to make each chapter self-contained, we have been willing to accept that some motifs may have to be discussed more than once. In the chapters on the meditations for the specific professions, we have reproduced the full text of each and largely refrained from page references. Accordingly some motifs in the text of other chapters are also repeatedly taken up so that they are more easily readable and comprehensible in themselves.

We would like to thank all our colleagues and co-workers who encouraged us to undertake this new edition. Very warm thanks are also due to our editor Ute E. Fischer and the Verlag am Goetheanum for its support.

For the International Coordination of Anthroposophic Medicine / IKAM

Michaela Glöckler and Rolf Heine
Medical Section at the Goetheanum
St John’s Tide 2015

Foreword to the first edition

The editors – representing the International Coordination of Anthroposophic Medicine/IKAM – intend the following accounts to be a situation analysis of the current stage of development of the anthroposophic medical movement.

Rolf Heine – coordinator for nursing in IKAM – drafted the organogram of the anthroposophic medical movement. Colleagues from all over the world commented on this draft; the IKAM collegium subsequently worked further on it and agreed its final form.

Even if the initial intention was to undertake this work solely for internal use, it soon became apparent that it might be of interest for other professional movements working in a manner inspired by anthroposophy. For those entrusted with leadership and management tasks in the various realms of anthroposophical cultural work draw on the same sources of inspiration.

We therefore decided to publish this work, also in view of the 150th anniversary of Rudolf Steiner's birth. Steiner's life work not only comprises his books and published lectures, it also contains a social edifice, an organogram for an internationally collaborating initiative community which endeavours to bring spirituality into the fields of research, training, professional and personal life. Our aim here is to make it visible through the example of the anthroposophic medical movement. We have therefore also included brief contributions on meditative work in professional practice. We likewise decided to revise and adapt the chapters on the Medical Section within the School of Spiritual Science from the Goetheanum brochure[2] for this purpose.

We hope this booklet will help its readers to recognise Rudolf Steiner's importance as the inaugurator of modes of work in which the peace-endowing principles of spiritual guidance constructively complement the necessities of today's world of work.

We would like to take this opportunity to thank everyone warmly who helped to set this publication on its way.

We look forward to receiving comments and suggestions.

Michaela Glöckler and Rolf Heine
Medical Section at the Goetheanum
Easter 2010

Introduction – Towards a leadership culture with "heart"

Michaela Glöckler

The anthroposophic medical movement, as one of the anthroposophical cultural initiatives, is a child of the twentieth century. Founded by the Austrian philosopher and anthroposophist Rudolf Steiner Ph. D. (1861 – 1925) and the Dutch physician Dr med. Ita Maria Wegman (1876 – 1943), it introduces anthroposophical insights regarding the spiritual nature of the self and the world into the field of medicine. In other words, it combines academic scientific medicine with the results obtained by anthroposophy.[3]

In social terms, the anthroposophic medical movement participates in the destiny of the Anthroposophical Society as well as in the impulses of the general anthroposophical movement inaugurated by Steiner which has its centre in the School of Spiritual Science in Dornach, Switzerland.

In 1923/24 Steiner refounded and reorganised the Anthroposophical Society at a conference held during the Christmas period – which is why it is referred to as the Christmas Conference – and transferred its headquarters from Germany to Switzerland. He tasked the newly founded society with supporting the School of Spiritual Science and established the different specialist sections which were to put anthroposophy into practice and enable it to take substantive effect. Thus a definitive point of departure was created for various professional movements inspired by anthroposophical thinking. On the other hand this also made it possible to embed in these professional movements an accompanying leadership culture.

For in establishing the specialist sections, Rudolf Steiner simultaneously entrusted the heads of these sections with the task of "leading the various branches of the anthroposophical movement".[4] The question remained open, however, as to what he understood leadership to mean. Furthermore, the question arises today as to the extent to which his original conception corresponds to what is needed to meet the demands of a modern leadership culture.

Why, in developing the Anthroposophical Society and the connected School of Spiritual Science, did Steiner not adhere rigorously to the democratic rules common in associations, thus risking being misunderstood or regarded as the founder of a rather backward-looking, hierarchically led community?

In the case of the anthroposophic medical movement, what arguments might there be, for instance, in favour of founding an internationally active, "worldwide umbrella association for anthroposophic medical initiatives and professional associations" that is led and controlled following the principles of direct democracy? It is clear that a large professional movement with a public profile requires organisational structures and leadership. But which form is the most suitable and would correspond to the intentions of the founders?

The question as to the conditions which best enable a professional movement which draws on spiritual inspiration to develop is a new one and it is relevant not only for anthroposophic medical work. It would seem natural either to take a lead from the Christmas Conference statutes conceived by Steiner – even though he himself was not able to test the fruitfulness of the leadership forms inherent within them due to his premature death – or develop possible new types of orientation.

However enthusiastic one might feel about testing and as far as possible realising such forms of work, suggested but not yet implemented by Steiner, it is equally clear that this will only succeed if the people working in the anthroposophic medical movement want it.

This was the situation when Michaela Glöckler – in close discussion with, and supported by the executive council of the Society of Anthroposophic Physicians in Germany and subsequently by the International Council of Anthroposophic Medical Associations – assumed responsibility for the leadership of the Medical Section at the Goetheanum in 1988. There was a strong will amongst the group of anthroposophic physicians to shape the continuation of the work in inner connection with the Goetheanum and its founding intentions. But it was an unresolved question as to how to make Steiner's social edifice of the School of Spiritual Science, its Sections and the Anthroposophical Society accessible in the daily work of this professional movement.

The accounts compiled here show what we have achieved so far and the extent to which the forms of work which Steiner proposed and laid down in ideal terms have proven to be inspiring, serviceable and practicable for the development of sustaining social structures in the anthroposophic medical movement.

Up to now we have found to be true what Marie Steiner wrote in 1944 in the foreword to the publication about the Christmas Conference mentioned above:

"The whole scope of negotiations is for us a path of schooling in matters concerning the management of meetings and dealing with the problems of the Society. [...] There is an endeavour at work to accomplish worldly things in a practical and purposeful way yet at the same time to subject them to the will of wise cosmic guidance. By this means daily matters are elevated to the sphere of spiritual goals and higher necessities."[5]

In saying this, Marie Steiner demonstrated how the modes of work conceived by Steiner remain capable of realisation and offer continuing inspiration. If we seek modes of work through which daily obligations and practical needs can be subjected to "wise cosmic guidance" – that is, to an inner, spiritual guidance available to all those involved – then leadership acquires the dimension of "spiritual leadership". But this is required when the further development of a professional movement is at stake which obtains its orientation from spiritual values and goals. Indeed, which experiences the latter as the guiding element.

What first began as "Anthroposophic Medicine" in 1921 in a small "Clinical and Therapeutic Institute" in Arlesheim has meanwhile become an autonomous form of therapy.[6] This gratifying development not only encompasses the work of physicians, including specialisations, but also nursing, physiotherapy, pharmacy, psychotherapy, special needs education, art therapy, eurythmy therapy and so forth.

Since 1986, a worldwide network of collaborating professionals has gradually formed within the anthroposophic medical movement. The reason for this development was increasing regulation of public health, both nationally and in the context of the European Union. To begin with it brought together physicians, manufacturers and consumers for regular discussions in the Filder Clinic near Stuttgart. But it soon became clear that other specialist fields also sought and needed collaboration.

While it is true that the anthroposophic medical movement so far has developed neither on the basis of strategic considerations nor through "central organisation" – from the beginning it was mostly entirely independent individual initiatives which expanded anthroposophic medicine worldwide – it is equally true that if further development is to thrive it needs exchange of experiences, mutual agreement and coordination. But what will a mode of coordination look like which not only acknowledges and promotes autonomy for initiatives by enterprising individuals as well as groups and associations but at the same time also coordinates and thus "leads" them?

Steiner's idea of leadership according to the model of the heart function (see page 46 ff.) connects these otherwise irreconcilable opposites. Because it is privileges of knowledge and information which give a "head-oriented", elitist leadership its typical character. "Hand-and-foot" oriented leadership, on the other hand, is marked by the centralised handling of financial and administrative resources. In contrast, leadership based on the model of the heart function supplies the whole organism with first-hand information. It decentralises money and administration and supports the development of various areas of responsibility in entrepreneurial self-governance (see page 76 ff.). It is based on mutual perception and impulse-giving, along with trust and conscious relinquishing of power. It promotes initiative and autonomy in those who are "led" as much as it does commitment and a proactive attitude towards the leaders' core concerns.

Correspondingly, the heart idea is a key concept in Steiner's idea of the individually and autonomously led sections in the School of Spiritual Science with simultaneous collegial overall responsibility for the School and the anthroposophical movement. The same thing applies analogously in IKAM: the international collegium of coordinators (see pages 58 ff., 65 ff., 76 ff., 87 ff.) corresponds to the collegium of section heads in the School of Spiritual Science. Each coordinator is individually responsible for "their" department of the anthroposophic medical movement, where feasible also to the extent of procuring the necessary financial and administrative resources. In joint responsibility for the whole movement, however, they sit side by side with the sections heads at the Goetheanum and together look beyond their own concerns into a wider, common field of tasks.

Anyone who has read this far might be thinking: how can such an ideal of leadership function in reality? Who is "mature" enough to want something like this, or to further its realisation? There is a simple answer: anyone who reflects on questions of leadership soon discovers the forward-looking character of Steiner's approach to self-governance which combines individual initiative with shared responsibility for the whole. The only question is whether we want to work in this way and how we can learn to do so.

The experience in the anthroposophic medical movement so far is reminiscent of the saying: "Those who want to, find ways; those who don't, find reasons." And: "Those who want to, are guided by the success of their work and human relationships. They learn from life and happily also from mistakes."

The following contributions show the manner in which it has so far been possible in the anthroposophic medical movement to realise Steiner's intentions with regard to leadership and what the consequences have been for its workflows.

Michaela Glöckler

The founding intentions and work of the Medical Section at the Goetheanum

Michaela Glöckler

Impulses which do not build on egoism

The tasks of the School of Spiritual Science, and with it also its Medical Section, are rooted in what Rudolf Steiner called the "spiritual injection" into the rising tides of materialism in the last third of the nineteenth century. These "rising tides of materialism" brought not only technical progress and material wealth for one part of humanity but also unspeakably aggravated social misery for another part.

Before the First World War, Rudolf Steiner's response to that social misery was the laying of the foundation stone of the first Goetheanum in 1913 as a school for conquering materialism in science and practical life. After the War, it was the foundation of the first Waldorf school in Stuttgart in 1919 at the request of the owner of the "Waldorf Astoria" cigarette factory, Emil Molt. Steiner thereby laid the foundations for a form of education "which does not build on egoism".[7]

In 1921 there followed the establishment of the first Clinical and Therapeutic Institute in Arlesheim and Stuttgart at the initiative of Ita Wegman and the group of physicians associated with Otto Palmer (1867 – 1945). This too was about the impulse of selflessness, of "caring morality" in medicine. Indeed, Steiner even described the nature of a spiritual medicine as "the most wonderful tool for an education to selflessness".[8] In 1922 the Christian Community was founded by a group of theologians who were seeking the spiritually awake connection with the stream of revelation of Christian salvation and asked Rudolf Steiner to help them in this.

In 1923/24 Steiner himself then decided to take on the leadership of the Anthroposophical Society as a large international organisation to support anthroposophical initiatives; he did the same with the Goetheanum whose School of Spiritual Science he gave the task of being a centre for all these endeavours to infuse professional life with spirit. He also set up sections for art, science and agriculture, mathematics and astronomy, social sciences as well as for the spiritual striving of youth and general anthroposophical work. The previously existing specialist fields of education and medicine were integrated into the School and the process of integrating the movement for spiritual renewal and the Christian Community also conceptually prepared.

Rudolf Steiner appointed co-workers to head these sections in the School of Spiritual Science who were willing to take the path of selfless devotion to the impulses coming from the spiritual world. To support this willingness, he set up in the General Anthroposophical Section a meditative course in the form of the so-called First Class of the School of Spiritual Science. This consisted of 19 situational meditations and the associated explanations through which it is possible to embark on the path out of the here-and-now of ordinary conventional everyday consciousness to the threshold of the spiritual world, and beyond that to the spiritual wellspring of existence.[9]

This path leads from "self"-referential self-knowledge to a form of self-knowledge through which it is possible to experience oneself working in accordance with the will of God and selflessly in his service. Rudolf Steiner once put what he understood this to mean concisely in the following words: "True meditation, however, is the fulfilment of the spiritual will which bears the spirit of our time within it. Where such meditation is practised, it is possible for a spiritual power to intervene in events on earth. Spiritual worlds want to intervene in events on earth today but they can only do so if the space for that is created through human meditation. Through this something like a gap is created in the physical field which spiritual beings and their actions can enter."[10]

It is not, therefore, surprising that he told the 800 members attending the Christmas Conference, which was concerned with outlining the tasks connected with the overall impulse of the Goetheanum as the School of Spiritual Science and headquarters of the Anthroposophical Society: "A revelation of the spirit was opened up for humanity. And not from any arbitrary earthly consideration but through a vision of the sublime pictures given out of the spiritual world as a modern revelation for the spiritual life of humanity – from this flowed the impulse for the anthroposophical movement. This anthroposophical movement is not an act of service to the earth, this anthroposophical movement in its totality and in all its details is a service to divine beings, a service to God. And we create the right mood for it when we see it in all its wholeness as such a service to God."[11]

This makes clear that the founding of the Goetheanum as an independent school for anthroposophy was an initiative with which Rudolf Steiner intended to facilitate practical divine service in the anthroposophically-inspired professional fields. The cause for this initiative was Ita Wegman's question about the renewal of ancient spiritual mystery medicine in contemporary form (see page 34 ff.).

It represented a mighty cultural paradigm change. It was no longer to be the case – as is normal today – that only representatives of the clergy were to engage in divine service. On the contrary, every person working in a profession was to be empowered to ask themselves to what extent they wanted and were able to feel themselves responsible in their actions towards a real, divine-spiritual world. Spirituality, the search for a spiritual path and identity is not just a matter for the religious professions but lives today as a longing in every human being, even if often unconsciously.

With such an endeavour, Steiner was the first in the modern era to link back to this most ancient of mystery traditions. "Mysterion" translated from the Greek means "secret". It stood for initiation rites which were kept secret because they were dangerous without special training and preparation. In contrast, the term for initiation in Christianity is "Apokalypsis", i.e. unveiling, disclosure, revelation. Spiritual knowledge for everyone who seeks it in accordance with the saying in St John's Gospel which is addressed to every thinking person: "And ye shall know the truth, and the truth shall make you free" (John 8:32). Steiner and his co-workers conceived of the Goetheanum as a place which was to enable such seeking and finding in the present time so that every person who wanted to could find the appropriate "path of initiation" for their profession in order to serve the goals which they had recognised for themselves and for which they were willing to bear responsibility.

Steiner put it as follows: "Since the School of Spiritual Science cannot be a college or university in the normal sense, it will not attempt to compete with these in any way or be a substitute for them. What can be found at the Goetheanum, however, which is not to be found at ordinary universities, is esoteric deepening of knowledge. People will be able to receive there something that the soul seeks in its quest for knowledge. This quest for knowledge can be something universally human. The General Section will exist for those who only have this universally human need to find the paths of the soul towards the world of spirit. It will form an 'esoteric school' for them. The other sections will endeavour to indicate paths where those who wish to orient their lives in accordance with a specific scientific, artistic or other way can do so. Thus every seeking human being will find at the 'Goetheanum School' what they wish to strive for, depending on the particular circumstances of their life. In other words, the School does not aim to be a purely academic institution, but a purely human one; but at the same time it should be able to fully engage with the esoteric needs of the scientist and the artist."[12]

This gives rise to a number of questions which we will deal with below:

- What is the position of the "Christian impulse" of anthroposophy in global transculturality?
- What is the "universally human" spiritual approach of anthroposophy?
- How can the Goetheanum in reality be the centre of an international and multicultural place of renewal of the mysteries?
- Was it not precisely a feature of the ancient mysteries that they were very much tied to peoples and traditions?
- How can we conceive of an "international", "transcultural", "universally human" mystery system?

Let me give a personal response to these questions. Because every single person is called upon today to say how their search along the path relates to the search of their fellow human beings. Without such questions, without a real interest in understanding the paths of the others, there can be no development of the active tolerance and capacity for peace which is essential for the humanisation process of humanity.

The father of a pupil in Beijing once opened my eyes to the full consequences of these issues when I wanted to know why he had entrusted his son to a Waldorf school which had only been established a few years previously. He told me: I don't know much about anthroposophy yet – but what I have understood of it and experience in the attitude and endeavour of children and teachers shows me that this way of developmentally oriented thinking and action will help us in China today to reconnect with our ancient spiritual roots, but in a new form. I subsequently encountered this view repeatedly during my visits to other cities in China.

Modern materialism – which Rudolf Steiner often characterised as a phenomenon of fear in the soul and spiritual illness – has become a global phenomenon today. It has turned the striving for material profit, for standing and outer prestige, into the dominant cultural quality. But once this has been achieved to a certain extent, it becomes obvious that such striving is insufficient also to nourish human beings in their soul and spirit and enable them to keep themselves healthy even when the circumstances of life are painful and unhappy.

Materialism has no "inner power" which could give a goal and direction to human life. But the maintenance of physical and mental health requires above all the possibility of understanding our own biography as a "school of life" and processing the events of our life in a way that gives meaning to it.

Such inner competence and willingness to develop must be awoken through education and role models. Otherwise there is a danger of despairing, burning out or falling prey to inner void. Hence access to spirituality is needed today which can build a bridge between materialistic science and spiritual experience. And because this is precisely what anthroposophy endeavours to do, it can build such a bridge. Because its instrument is human thinking which is, on the one hand, the basis of academic research and can, on the other hand, be developed to understand and identify spiritual connections.

Thinking, and with it philosophy, can describe the values

which are typical of all spiritual and religious systems. It was the German philosopher Karl Jaspers (1883 – 1969) who coined the term "axial age". He understood this to be the period between 800 and 200 BC in which individual thinking developed in the four great cultural regions on earth and manifested historically in great personalities.

All the conceptions and value systems which are familiar to humanity today started in this period: in China Laozi and Confucius were at work, teaching the path of the development of ideas which is guided by clear ethical values such as love, frugality, humility, tolerance and the harmonious order of things and of the state, which is valid to the present day. In India the comprehensive teaching of empathy and love appeared with Siddhartha Gautama Buddha and along with that a conscious dealing with the concept of reincarnation and the development of destiny. In the Middle East – Hebrews and Persians – the Biblical prophets appeared, as did Zarathustra with the concept of the battle between good and evil.

In the West, in contrast, Greek philosophy started with the early natural philosophers and went on to Socrates, Plato and Aristotle, determining the ethical and philosophical foundation of the European western world to the present day with the cardinal virtues of justice, temperance, courage, wisdom and devoutness standing under the control of reason and the Logos. We encounter such a foundation of human developmental perspectives also in Rudolf Steiner's anthroposophy. It builds on German Idealism (Fichte, Hegel, Schelling, Schiller, Goethe) with its rigorous focus on individual development guided by the central values of humanity in the form of truthfulness, love and freedom.

Ultimately all four cultural regions are concerned with mighty impulses of humanisation, the development of the I, the individual personality by means of the thinking, and the wish to unite personally with ethical values and ideals. Anthroposophy forms no exception to this. But it contributes to these great value systems, which are very similar to one another in their innermost substance, the possibility of realisation in everyday life, the relationship with practical life in all its details. Its path of schooling is practice-oriented through and through.

Anthroposophy is not just about becoming an ethically more perfect person. It teaches that every spiritual insight, every inner virtue only leads to good if it becomes truly mirrored in life. Anthroposophy is ultimately only concerned with applying the lessons of life, with serving humanity as a whole. Hence its name: "anthropos", translated from the Greek, means "human being" and "sophia" means "wisdom". So it may rightly be said: anthroposophy does not contribute any new additional values to the ones formulated during the axial period. But it shows an inner path to these values which leads directly into practical life and healthfully supplements materialistic science, which itself cannot develop any ethics, and makes it comprehensible at a deeper level.

In this way the gap is bridged which has opened up between the "belief and trust" in a spiritual world and the "knowledge about things" of modern science. Anthroposophy thus sees itself as a science of the spirit. It is not a matter of belief or religion. On the contrary, Rudolf Steiner demanded of his pupils: "You should not believe what I say but think it through."[13] That is why there are people worldwide who implement initiatives out of anthroposophy in the fields of agriculture, education, art and medicine completely independently of their religion or meditative practice, or the spiritual orientation to which they belong.

An anthroposophical physician in India once told me that anthroposophy had helped her to understand her ancient religion of Hinduism better, which is why she was now able to appreciate it again profoundly. An anthroposophical architect in Japan told me the same thing with regard to Buddhism which he practised. And in Egypt, in the Islamic cultural sphere, the anthroposophical pioneer and winner of the Alternative Nobel Prize, Ibrahim Abouleish, said it with regard to the wisdom of the Koran and the religion of Islam, to which he feels spiritually committed.

I feel the same way about Christianity. This religion only became truly accessible for me with the help of anthroposophical spiritual science. These examples show that modern human beings want to obtain understanding – including of their beliefs – otherwise they feel uncomfortable. It is the mission of anthroposophy to make a consistent contribution to the success of such an understanding. Since every person seeks and goes their own path in complete freedom, and the foundation of a thinking comprehension is common to all people, its study also provides the potential for the so necessary all-inclusive tolerance and acceptance of those who think differently from us.

Because then we understand and respect why other people think in different ways. The strength of anthroposophy lies not just in its "knowledge" – everyone acquires that in their own way. Its strength rests above all in the possibility of implementing what has been learnt. Hence "doing anthroposophy" is also the key word around which everything revolved at the Christmas Conference and which the Goetheanum with its facilities wants to serve.

The threshold to the spiritual world

As early as in a public lecture on 1 May 1919 in Stuttgart, Rudolf Steiner set out the necessity of having a clear understanding that the thresholds of birth and death are transitions into spiritual forms of existence of human beings to which our life on earth and in time also has a direct relationship.[14] He explained that happiness in life and the capacity to withstand crises are dependent on the extent to which a person is aware of this fact. Because those who live in the awareness that the spiritual world – in the form of life after death and before birth – actually exists, develop different values and perspectives on earthly life.

They learn to live daily life with more mindfulness in every respect and to acknowledge responsibility for their own actions to themselves and their guiding spirit. If we do not become aware of this fact, we lose insight into the meaning and purpose of life, as well as into the precious nature of every moment granted to us to develop ourselves and work for others.

Cultivating "threshold consciousness", on the other hand, in professional and social life awakens each person's experience of meaning and sense of responsibility regarding the developmental context in which they stand; it gives life value and orientation. At the same time much is also "unveiled" in the sense of the "apocalypse" referred to previously. Consciously approaching the threshold to the spiritual world is a serious matter – as is the search for truth and self-knowledge as forms of expression of such proximity to the threshold.[15]

In the esoteric tradition, the three decisive steps for individually preparing the conscious crossing of the threshold are described in images as the trials by fire, water and air.[16] Formerly, at the time of the ancient mysteries, these trials or tests could only be undergone in the form of initiation rituals in a temple. Today the inner and outer circumstances in the lives of most people are such that life itself requires such trials. Life has become a mystery whose meaning and developmental perspectives have to be uncovered. The initiation experiences "through the trials of life" which become possible as a result relate to our cognitive, feeling and will life.

Trial of fire: in the fire of honest knowledge of ourselves and the world, the self-deception with which we unconsciously want to protect ourselves and others from uncomfortable truths is burned away.

Trial by water: in the crisis of trust which very often follows a severe disappointment in ourselves or another person, we experience the quality of the trial by water in which "nothing supports us any longer". In the face of the deep uncertainty associated with this, the falling away of acceptance, support and encouragement from within and without, we can only develop further in a healthy way by deriving our motives for action entirely from within ourselves and out of the matter at hand. Personal sympathies can and must fall silent here. The love for an action rooted solely in the matter at hand itself sustains us in such a situation, even if we are otherwise floundering.

Trial by air: the quality of the trial by air, in contrast, concerns a capacity which the modern human being especially needs if they wish to act in a culturally creative and healing way. Here we must not only educate ourselves to be truthful to ourselves and others (the fire trial process) and develop a capacity for human understanding or love (the water trial process). This requires in particular the capacity for moral intuition,[17] that is to say, the ability to make the right decision. This demands courage, tolerance and an unconditional love of freedom without which action with true presence of mind is not possible.

These three new ways of handling thinking, feeling and volition – even if we initially only practice them in a tentative way – turn social life into a developmental space for all. But at the same time they are also the capacities or attitudes towards life that connect the spiritual and sensory worlds and facilitate a conscious crossing of the threshold to the spiritual world.

Moral techniques for social engagement

In the face of the social deficiencies that are so commonly experienced today, it is important to detail the social skills that are required:

- In the spiritual and cultural sphere we need to develop individualism and personal commitment – what one might call spiritual entrepreneurship.
- In the sphere of rights we need clear structures for reaching agreements and opportunities to reflect on the forms of work in which we are embedded so that we can optimise them for the benefit of all.
- In the economic and social sphere the primary need is for a culture of acknowledgement of what is achieved, of what each individual can contribute with their specific gifts and capacities.

When these three primary needs of modern human beings are taken into account, we can respond to the "difficulties" in social life in a constructive way. The creative development of all can replace the chaotic drifting apart of individual intention. In order to provide inner orientation in this respect, Steiner outlined three possible forms of community building during the Christmas Conference on 27 December 1923 – two with a horizontal structure and one that vertically crosses and connects them.[18]

The working forms characterised by horizontal lines are those of the General Anthroposophical Society and the School of Spiritual Science with its three classes (see sketch: I, II, III, next page) of which Steiner himself was only able to establish the First Class in its first division. The "vertical" community building in the

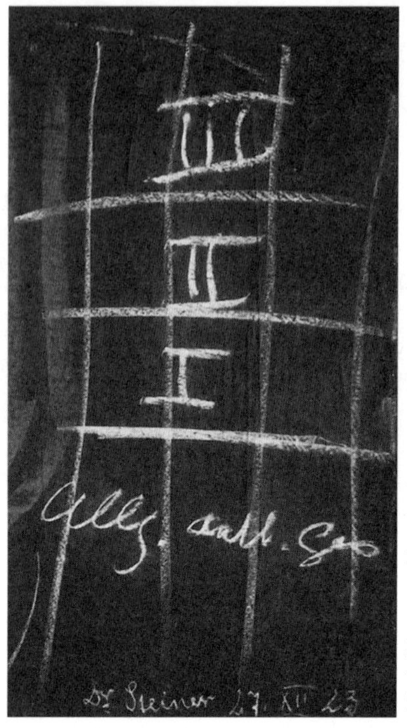

Rudolf Steiner's sketch, explained at the Christmas Conference of 1923/24 to clarify the working forms of the Anthroposophical Society, School of Spiritual Science and the Sections

context of the sections is rooted in an inner attitude to accomplish daily work out of spiritual responsibility. This requires the autonomy and fraternal stance that can be learned in the forms of work of the Anthroposophical Society and the School.

In the statutes of the General Anthroposophical Society as conceived by Steiner, its working forms are entirely founded on each individual's initiative.[19] Every member is accorded the autonomous right to join a working group or to form a group with others that has a local or thematic focus.[20]

In the School of Spiritual Science, on the other hand, there are no statutes describing the rights and duties of members. Steiner calls this the "soul of the Anthroposophical Society".[21] To become a member of the School, no admission test is required, no certificate of competence as is otherwise normal for higher education institutions. Nor is any members' contribution stipulated, as is the case in the Anthroposophical Society. On the contrary, the entry requirements are purely human and moral qualities, three developmental conditions which a person affirms with a binding commitment both to themselves and to the School collegium – the group of section leaders – that they will seek to fulfil them:

1. To pursue the anthroposophical path of development independently and with commitment.[22]
2. To "stay connected" with the other School members.[23]
3. To be a representative of the anthroposophical cultural impulse "in all details of life".[24]

These three conditions give each individual a clear orientation and create the coherence necessary for forming working contexts, or "communities of free spirits". In the context of these reflections it also becomes clear that it is these three conditions through which the "renewal of the mysteries" becomes possible. The whole of the human being is involved: the thinking in the individual search for the path; the feeling in knowing oneself connected in spiritual brotherly and sisterly love with the others; and the will in representing what we have chosen to pursue. In his "Letters to Members 1924" Rudolf Steiner describes these three conditions implicitly and explicitly as a social path of schooling to make anthroposophy most effective individually and communally.[25]

It is also an interesting feature that in giving mandates and assignments, Rudolf Steiner always kept to individuals. When collegial structures came into play, then always in such a way that the holders of individual responsibilities were called upon to work together jointly on a higher level – both in the leadership of the branches and groups of the Anthroposophical Society and in the collegium of the School. Anthroposophical work was to be characterised by an "esoteric trait": "The only thing that can establish and maintain the Anthroposophical Society in an esoteric sense is what is present as real human relationships. Thus in the future everything has to be built on real human relationships in the widest sense, on concrete and not on abstract spiritual life."[26]

This makes clear what we can take "esotericism" and "esoteric" to mean in a concrete sense: the spirituality of life in the diversity of its interactions and relations as well as the spirituality of human relationships when they are "real". In a Christian sense this is about the principle: "For where two or three are gathered together in my name, there am I in the midst of them" (Matthew 18:20). Each person works individually on their own responsibility and is at the same time interested in the contribution of the others. This creates the necessary permeability for those things which can be realised through the community as a higher commission from and will of the spiritual world.

The Raphael Imagination as the inspiration for medical and therapeutic action

On 7 October 1923, Rudolf Steiner in the context of his lectures on the four seasons – and in preparation for the Christmas Conference – developed the Raphael Imagination as a source of inspiration for the Easter festival: the Risen Christ walking and holding the balance between Lucifer and Ahriman – just as it is also expressed in Rudolf Steiner's wooden sculpture. Raphael is the archangel whose existence is wholly in the service of these balance-creating forces of the Risen Christ. The Dutch psychiatrist, special needs teacher and specialist in organisational development, Bernard Lievegoed, in 1982 wrote the appeal in looking up to Raphael:[27]

Raphael!

Brother of humanity –
who stands beside us
giving us courage
where we want to act to heal –
where we want to bring development
back into destiny in stalemate.

Who, to redeem,
makes earth's darkness
flare up
in light and warmth
around his staff.

Help us –
because we too want to
transform human darkness
and let human light and warmth
flare up in human hearts.

The unceasing struggle for balance, for the creation of harmony, is at the same time the wellspring of health:

> physically in the self-regulation of the organism,
> psychologically in the will for self-education,
> spiritually in the work to guide the I, as the core of our being, to an awareness of its freedom and thus to the source of the balance-creating activity in human beings.

This is the individual aspect of health. The social aspect concerns the creation of harmony in the karmic relationships between people on earth and the essence of healing in the sense that problematic relationships become comprehensible and thus accessible to "healing through destiny". In addition there is the human aspect. Each person is part of humanity as a whole and thus contributes through their individual and social behaviour to the wellbeing or misery of this great developmental context.

Accordingly Raphael is a concealed archangel. We know much less about him than about Gabriel or Michael. It is all the more surprising, then, that Goethe in the Prologue in Heaven of his *Faust* has Raphael speak first, and thus names the primal ground of divine harmony and of the "cosmic health" predisposed in all Creation which underlies every event, however tragic it might be.

Thus the words of Raphael resound in the Prologue in Heaven:

The sun sings out as it has always
Competing with its brother spheres,
And on its predetermined journey
Completes its course with thunderous peals.
Its aspect gives the angels power,
Though none may fathom all its ways;
The lofty works beyond conception
Glorious as on the primal day.

(*Goethe, Faust I*)

Turning to this healthy element in the human being and trusting it unshakably is the most important Raphaelic virtue from which the "courage to heal", which Steiner so powerfully urged physicians to have,[28] is fed.

Ita Wegman sensed this secret, she had the courage to heal and the "invincible will of karma".[29] Hence she was also able to ask the question about a renewal of the medical mysteries. Notes she made about this – in her typical Dutch-German writing style – have been preserved. They were written in 1936, one year after the general meeting of the Anthroposophical Society whose members dismissed her and her colleague Elisabeth Vreede from the executive council and expelled many members from the Society who were friends of Ita Wegman. The tragedy associated with this can be heard in her words.

We reproduce notes below which she wrote down in preparation of a medical conference in her Clinical and Therapeutic Institute in Arlesheim:[30] "[There were] two questions which I asked Dr Steiner, I can even specify the time very precisely when I made them. The first question in Britain after Penmaenmawr / summer school: why is the mystery part in medicine not given greater prominence and cast into a form? Why do the medical courses have to be held in such an intellectual way? It had to be like that, Dr Steiner says, because the conditions for the other are not yet given. It is very important that you ask this question. In October/November 1923 he then held the many mystery lectures, the Michael, Christmas, Easter, St John's Tide Imagination lectures in which the cosmic art of healing was discussed. The Christmas Conference was founded, new life blossomed in the Anthroposophical Society. And a real start was made in giving medicine a new form. Let me remind you of the lectures given to the young medics. The mystery principle is that we learn to think in a pictorial way, that the events in the whole cosmos are absorbed in images, thus also healing in the cosmos and healing in the microcosm which is only an image of the macrocosmic. The images then have to be brought together in meditations.

My second question to Dr Steiner was shortly before he fell ill in September 1924. I asked: is it not possible to found a medical mystery school? Rudolf Steiner's response was: It is not that simple, it must be wanted by the spiritual world and there have to be people who want to receive it. A few days later he told me that he had asked the Mercury-Raphael spirit and had received an affirmative answer. He had been assigned the task of renewing old traditions which had once taken place in holy, ancient sites under the leadership of Mercury-Raphael. My task was to seek spirit-borne human souls who had a feel for such work and were willing to hear Raphael's words.

We consequently then made a very small beginning. In this way the seed was planted for a Raphael school.

My dear friends, that was significant. The things which were healing principles in the various mysteries, brought together in a school. Michael and Raphael working together!

Unfortunately it was not to be, one could literally feel the resistance of the earth. Earth and human beings did not want such immense spirituality yet. Dr Steiner then left his work on earth of his own volition, his illness was just Maya. And people were left on their own, lapsed into the bad old ways of seeing everything intellectually and judging it rationally. The Anthroposophical Society was shaken to its foundations. Karmic relationships were thrown off balance. People were not yet mature enough to receive so much spirituality or also – this is the positive part in all the arguing and fighting – that retarding forces which are also often necessary, having some idea that the maturity was not yet there, resisted the course of events in order to pre-empt spiritual imperfections in spiritual development. This is where we are.

... We have the longing for a mystery medicine. We cannot continue what was started just like that. We have to try to prepare ourselves again to awaken a spiritual memory in ourselves of what once existed in the mysteries. I am willing to do anything in my power to help in this.

Clarify who the Mercury-Raphael being is.

Michael helps human beings in their struggle to transform consciousness of nature into consciousness of self, to create [the latter]. Michael is here, the spiritual, the cosmic healer, acting on the head. Mercury-Raphael stands next to human beings, acting on the respiratory system. Just as Michael's flaming sword is made of cosmic iron and with this power fights against the nature-consciousness of human beings which is trying to rise up and conjures up self-consciousness (Notebook 57)."[31]

From the correspondence between the young physicians published by Peter Selg, we know the great extent to which the question was alive among the physicians as to what Rudolf Steiner and Ita Wegman expected of them and what medicine was truly about.[32]

One thing did and has become very clear in this: it is not enough to be a good physician or therapist – it requires simultaneously the development of sustainable communities of "spirit-borne human souls" who are willing also to work to create harmony in their destiny. Because most medical conditions which make a patient go to the doctor are rooted in a lack of harmony in the circumstances of destiny. Hence great possibilities of working in a healing way are also concealed in the formation of therapeutically active communities.

Rudolf Steiner made a start with such a community in September 1924. It happened during the Pastoral Medicine Course. He told the physicians present there in an address on 18 September: "Aspiring to such a source of activity here at the Goetheanum for medicine, that is the thinking and striving of the collaboration between Dr. Wegman and myself. And the purpose of what healers take away with them from the medical course in the Medical Section at the Goetheanum can really only lie in connecting with what is intended here to be the source, in the awareness of belonging together: a real feeling of belonging together with what is intended to take its starting point from the centre I have indicated.

And so I may say in conclusion particularly to you, my dear friends: seek for the way which in this sense represents the association of practising physicians. Seek the way to such an association. You will find it. And it will be our concern at the Goetheanum that you shall find it. That a first step should be taken in this direction has given Dr Wegman and me reason to make a start by giving an initial esoteric impulse in that an esoteric core has been established which can easily be extended; as I said, it can easily be extended but there are good reasons for it to consist to begin with of a number of medical practitioners who in turn have made the commitment which is necessary for esoteric medical work. This core consists of the medical practitioners: Dr Walter, Dr Bockholt, Dr Zeylmans, Dr Glas, Dr Schickler, Dr Knauer, Dr Kolisko." [...]

"It is this, after all, which is the best thing that the Goetheanum can do: finding people who are active outside in the world in the greatest variety of human activity and whose intentions are always an echo of what is said here at the Goetheanum and what it aims to do. If you do that in your field, then a bond of cohesiveness, a Goethean spirit will link you hearts and souls and we will see fruits keep arising for the benefit of humankind if you keep finding your way to the Goetheanum here. Because, after all, everything that is done here is always a fragment, a part, always starting capital to begin with. The more we can hope that it will provide motivation for individuals to take more and more of it away with them, the more the goal is achieved. This is what I ask you to take away with you and what I wanted to say to you. And with that let me conclude this course on pastoral medicine with a heartfelt greeting to you all."[33]

This community reconstituted itself after the Second World War and is known as the Easter or Raphael Group. A publication which describes the conditions under which it was founded and the development of its present forms of working is not yet available. The words which Rudolf Steiner spoke at its establishment have been preserved and were published in 1999.[34] They describe how Raphael turned to Rudolf Steiner and Ita Wegman, calling on them to renew ancient mystery traditions and to seek spirit-borne human souls who want to participate in this renewal. Accordingly, this book also wishes to make a contribution to bringing the Raphaelic quality in the work context of the anthroposophic medical movement to greater awareness and thus to make it more manageable.

Since Rudolf Steiner and Ita Wegman were connected by destiny in a relationship in which there was the greatest possible harmony, it was possible for the Raphaelic being to turn to and work with them. Even if the Raphael Group was founded as a purely medical group, it bears within it the intention of new medical ethics and practice which concerns the whole of the anthroposophic medical movement. The task is to work on forms of a "Raphaelic culture" in the way medicine is practised today.

Future work perspectives and the question as to the qualities of the Second and Third Classes of the School intended by Rudolf Steiner

The social structure of the anthroposophical movement, the Society and the School as described above shows how the social aspect of the anthroposophical cultural impulse as a whole was conceived, and how its diverse organs and working contexts can mutually and fruitfully interpenetrate one another. However, the question remains open as to what qualities and possibilities for work would have been added by the Second and Third Classes which are located in the second and third horizontal line of the sketch of 27 December 1923. This question is particularly crucial for the work of the sections, whose vertical structure crosses the levels of the classes which were intended by Steiner but no longer realised.

Since there are only a few oral and written indications and suggestions from Rudolf Steiner about the School's further development, views about this and attitudes relating to further work range from respectfully refraining from all further thoughts on the matter through to specific approaches to possible modes of work, such as the one presented below.[35] This latter one is based on the little that has been passed on, and on the above-named conditions for membership of the School (see page 31 ff.). The conditions testify to three very different competencies that must be developed if anthroposophical cultural work is to succeed. The first condition relates to the development of individual spiritual autonomy (individual competence). The second concerns the elaboration of social competence. The third conditions leads to a Christian and Rosicrucian attitude to life: placing everything we have learned in the service of life and human development.

The associated approach to work is furthermore rooted in the three great cultural impulses of science, art and religion which can be found in the basic orientation of the three classes.

Steiner not only entrusted Ita Wegman with the leadership of the Medical Section but also with the leadership of the First Class of the School. She took on the inner, spiritual task of overcoming materialism, which especially threatens the human being in academic medicine, and of learning how it is possible to introduce spirituality quite specifically even into the smallest actions of daily medical practice. Her goal was to make anthroposophy effective in all medical knowledge and procedures. The imaginations, words and symbols conveyed by Steiner in the First Class lessons show the way in which the profound insult to consciousness caused by prevailing scientific materialism can be overcome. This involves a path of inner schooling, the path of spiritual science, which focuses primarily on discovering truth (the fire trial process) and is not satisfied solely with principles such as practicability or reproducibility.

To outline the tasks connected with the work of the Second Class, it is helpful to examine the founding impulse[36] of the Society for the Theosophical Way of Life and Art[37] ("Gesellschaft für theosophische Art und Kunst"), which was launched in 1911, and the artistic work on the Mystery Dramas.[38] Here the focus is on developing spiritual and social capacities and skills, on the acquisition of social artistry, and on taking karma and the shaping of destiny seriously: people learn to work together with others who have different forms of destiny and orientation. What the Mystery Dramas show in their temple scenes applies here: how human destinies are wisely ordained, and how difficult it is for us to accept our destiny in full awareness without losing our orientation when social problems arise (the water trial process). These Mystery Dramas – but also Rudolf Steiner's "Letters to Members"[39] written in the last year of his life – offer rich study material for these qualities of work.

The few hints that we have relating to the work impulse of the Third Class suggest that it would involve religious rites in which, through real enactment, one could experience where the task of the anthroposophical movement stands in the context of humankind and the world, and how this task can most decisively be served. Thematically, the so-called Michael Letters (GA 26) point towards the prospect of developing substance and finding moral guidance. This can prepare for and support the reception of inspirations and intuitions from the spiritual world that accord with our time. The focus here is on the quality of the trial by air, on acting – with absolute presence of mind – "in the service of the time spirit Michael".[40]

Maintaining such future perspectives is particularly important in relation to the burning question of what we as contemporaries need to develop and work on in ourselves today so that we are not only sufficient to the moment but can also help to undertake the necessary preparations and set the strategic direction for cultural development in the fifth, sixth and seventh post-Atlantean epochs of evolution described by Steiner in his book *Occult Science* (GA 13).

It is clear that the work of the First Class is primarily devoted to meeting the cultural task that arises currently in this fifth cultural period: recognising and overcoming the destructive consequences of a materialistic science and worldview. The motifs of the Second Class are more connected with preparing the sixth cultural epoch, the era in which processes of community building and fraternity will determine culture. The outlined work impulses of the Third Class, in contrast, look ahead to the task of the seventh evolutionary period; here it will be necessary to transform the potential battle of all against all into a conscious integration of the individual into the whole of humanity. The Goetheanum thus sets itself in the tradition of the mystery sites of humanity not only to continue everyday life in the present out of past traditions but also in the service of what wants to develop in the future.

Rudolf Steiner spoke about the new mysteries as early as 1908 in a public lecture in Nuremberg which in contrast to the pre-Christian mysteries of wisdom are mysteries of the will:[41] it is therefore the core task of the School of Spiritual Science to find paths and forms of working for the various professions through which we can learn to realise such an existential involvement in the great tasks of humanity – right into the most ordinary duties and activities. It is a matter of making the qualities of "initiation through life" and through conscious individual schooling into the foundation of a civilisational development with future potential.[42]

Work and goals of the Medical Section

Why do human beings become ill? This is one of today's key questions. There is no area of social life unaffected by issues relating to pathology and therapy. Much of modern culture is conducive to illness: many people's attitude towards life and not infrequently their daily lives is determined by insecurity, anxiety, identity problems and violation of boundaries in the form of abuse and violence, both emotional and physical. Here it is all the more a necessity of our time to tap the sources of health, not just at a physical level but also, in particular, at a psychological and spiritual level. Above and beyond this, the Medical Section's very fundamental task is to seek out and illuminate therapeutic aspects involved in the work of the other sections too, and support them through collaboration.

To do so requires a new approach to the question of what pathology and therapy, the onset of illness and healing actually are. From this arises the Medical Section's core task. This consists of integrating anthroposophy as a spiritual science into medicine as a natural science and thus developing "the medical system of anthroposophy".[43] In this system the scientific and spiritual aspects of illness are elaborated in a way that reveals illness as the "physical imagination of spiritual life".[44] In other words, through its symptoms of illness the physical body reveals "unconscious self-knowledge – an unconscious initiation experience".[45] In one of his notebooks, Steiner outlines this self-encounter in illness as an unconscious encounter with the Guardian of the Threshold, that is to say, as an encounter with one's own very personal guidance of destiny:

At the threshold there stream
Senses' darkness and spirit's light
Into each other, creating illusion.
Illness is the reflection
Of this illusion
In illness lives the Guardian.
Conscious encounter in spirit,
Unconscious encounter in body.

Rudolf Steiner[46]

The spiritual view of the development of illness and its prevention indicated here opens up new aspects for diagnosis and therapy.

Health, in contrast, is shown to be the result of processes of education and self-education oriented to life and a person's own developmental goals. In the book *Extending Practical Medicine - Fundamental Principles based on the Science of the Spirit* (GA 27), jointly written by Ita Wegman and Rudolf Steiner, the authors highlight the path not only for establishing the foundations of anthroposophic medical research but also for training and therapeutic practice. The studies of substances and the human being developed there describe the connection between a person's life, soul and spirit in a way that makes clear how spirit and matter work together in the body. How, on the one hand, the soul-spiritual evolution of the human being is connected with types of substance formation and transformation in the body's processes; and on the other, how corresponding medicines undergo processes in their manufacturing which are similar to those which unfold in the human organism.[47]

Prevention, however, stands at the core of an anthroposophically-oriented health science – preventive work that stops the development of illness. Steiner called the preventive impulse "hygienic occultism" and the ability to prevent illness the hygienic occult ability.[48] What today we call primary prevention – preventing illness without any sign of it yet having appeared – is thinking wholly in line with hygienic occultism. Its focus is health-promoting, age-appropriate education and self-education. The theory of development and health it gives rise to underlies both the Waldorf education he founded and the path of self-development he proposed. It was his great concern to appeal to teachers and physicians to collaborate in the sense of the mystery traditions mentioned above, according to which it was known that the human being would fall ill if left solely to their own nature, and if not educated actively to greater humanity:

It was in ancient times,
That there lived in the souls of initiates
Powerfully the thought that
By nature every human being is sick.
And education was seen
As a healing process
Which, as they matured,
Gave children the health
To be complete human beings in life.

Rudolf Steiner[49]

In addition, it is not only the individual person who is vulnerable to illness and in need of healing but also the social organism of society. Here too Anthroposophic Medicine sees itself called upon to make a contribution. Because it would be healthy and of fundamental importance for spiritual and cultural life to become a locus of free initiative and personal self-development; for economic life to become oriented in a fraternal way to meet people's real needs; and if governments and legal systems created the laws necessary for this and for equality before the law.

The social reality we currently inhabit is by contrast pathological: currently the global economy, as a "free market economy", lives largely by the principle that is healthy for spiritual and cultural life: freedom. Cultural life at universities, in contrast, is currently adapted to clearly prescribed academic rules of play, watched over by the "scientific community". This points in the direction of fraternity or brotherliness. Between these a bureaucracy hypertrophying due to the overall pathological signature is attempting to rein in the risks to the biosphere resulting from scientific activities and the associated capitalist economy.

How can a Christian style of leadership succeed?

When on 1 January 1924, at the end of the Christmas Conference, Louis Werbeck expressed the thanks of the participants, he addressed Rudolf Steiner with the words: "You great, pure brother of humanity." He asked him for his "fatherly blessing" for the further work of the Anthroposophical Society. Steiner responded: "My dear friends, what has taken place here is something that I know I was allowed to say, for it was spoken with full responsibility and in looking upwards to the spirit who is there, and who should be and will be the spirit of the Goetheanum. In the name of this spirit I have allowed myself to speak things during these days that could not have been uttered so forcefully if not uttered looking upwards to the spirit of the Goetheanum. And so let me accept these thanks on behalf of the spirit of the Goetheanum, for whom we wish to exert ourselves and strive and work in the world."[50]

These words of Rudolf Steiner at the same time correspond to a new "principle of succession". In contrast to the "horizontal" succession which takes effect in the next in line through the laying on of hands or handing over the baton, etc., the principle of "vertical succession" is set up here in which Steiner included himself as the founder of anthroposophy. As little as he himself wished to receive thanks from others for his work, but passed it on to his source of inspiration in the spiritual world from which the "leadership" came, just as little did he value it when people cited his authority in terms of "horizontal succession" and did not speak "out of themselves".

A "Christian style of leadership" takes its lead from the Pauline attitude: "I live; yet not I, but Christ liveth in me."[51] But this is an attitude of "vertical succession". Anthroposophy aims

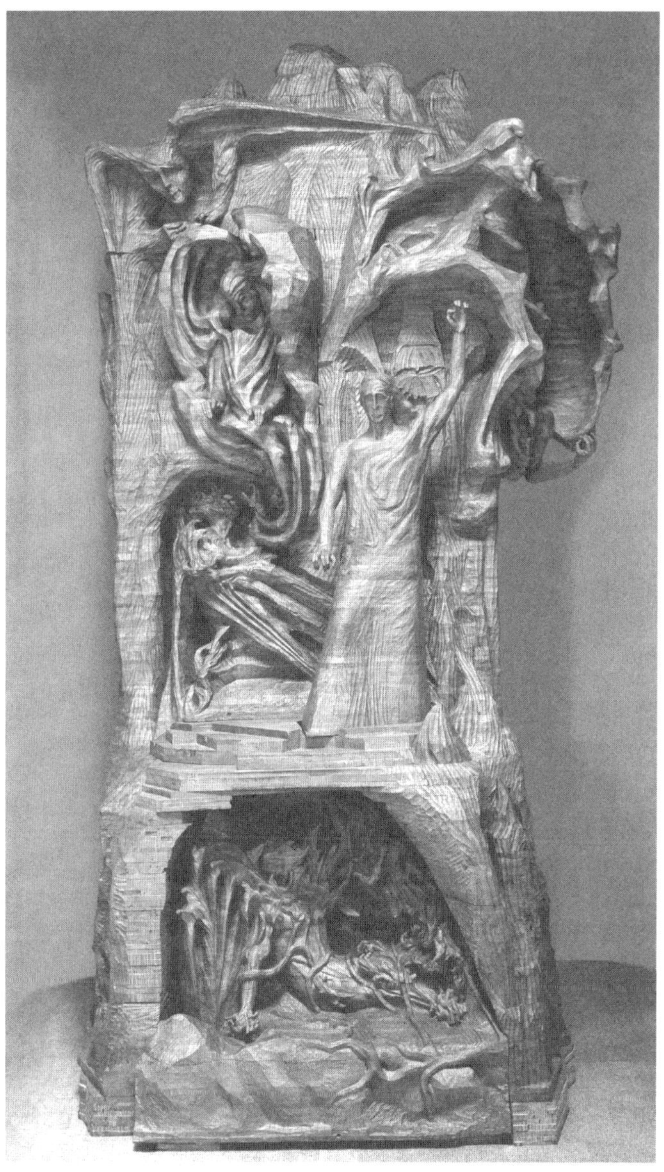

Christ as the representative of humanity between Lucifer and Ahriman, wooden sculpture by Rudolf Steiner (9.70 m).

to be a path to independent spiritual knowledge. In the field of science this is possible by spiritualising thinking, through meditation. In the artistic field through the creative handling of the artistic creative elements – building materials, forms, colours, tones, words, movements – in such a way that spiritual aspects can reveal themselves.[52] In practical life, in contrast, as much of what is specifically spiritually grasped and longed for in this way can be realised as the individual is able to accomplish through the nature of their work and way of life. Of these three forms of manifestation of spiritual realities, art has progressed the furthest. It can show images, revelations of "perfection".

It is hardly surprising, therefore, that Rudolf Steiner spoke often and in such a moving way about the nature of the Dornach building, and its central sculpture, the "Representative of Humanity". Over nine meters high, the statue shows Christ striding between the powers that seek to divert human beings from their path: Lucifer as the radiant spirit of an exaggerated opinion of oneself, and Ahriman as the power-conscious spirit of conformity and de-individualisation.

When building work on the first Goetheanum was starting, on occasion of the inauguration of the artists' studio on 17 June 1914, Steiner said: "But then, when all is ensouled by this spirit whom I wish to invoke with these words in this room this evening, when all the work that is undertaken across this hill is filled with this spirit of love, which at the same time is also always the spirit of authentic art, then from this hill and what stands here there will radiate out into the world the spirit of peace, the spirit of harmony, the spirit of love."[53]

The guiding image for the leadership culture of the Goetheanum, in particular for the Medical Section with its therapeutic task, is the heart function of the human being. The place in which the spirit of love referred to above has access. Steiner confirms this task everywhere in his work in formulations such as: "The inmost principle of anthroposophical endeavour is love for the human being."[54] "We can only make what we say and hear into the proper point of departure for the development of the anthroposophical cause if our heart's blood is capable of beating for it."[55] At the end of the Christmas Conference, his words sound like a Whitsun blessing: "And so, my dear friends, bear your warm hearts, in which you have laid the foundation stone for the Anthroposophical Society, bear these warm hearts into the world for strong, potent and healing work."[56] "And so the heartfelt ties which you can form with the Goetheanum will be something which, especially as physicians, can profoundly help you in the task you have really set yourselves."[57]

Steiner had a very clear perception of the connection between phenomena of social misery in his time – such as poverty, the upsurge of racism, abuses of power, and violence – and an education that was remote from the spirit, making it inadequate for developing freedom and responsibility. He regarded the social question as an educational one.

When the Waldorf School was founded, he proposed that education must have a therapeutic orientation – always serving individual development and focusing on the child's developing health. Thus the educational question becomes a medical-therapeutic one.

Ultimately, though, as Paracelsus saw it, the medical question is the question of the only true medicine, love. And so we come full circle: the social question is an educational one, the latter a medical one, and the medical question: what helps, what heals determines the attitude towards the social conditions.

The human heart perceives in a differentiated way – physiologically, emotionally and spiritually – what is happening in the organs and organ systems of the whole organism. It is from here that the whole receives its impulses and every single organ and function receives the heart's blood as necessary to meet individual requirements. It is in the heart that the particular potential, capacities, needs and stresses of individual organs are reflected, along with the needs of the whole.[58]

In the way the heart functions – its archetypal mediation between periphery and centre and between the polarities of the nervous and sensory system and the metabolic and limb system – it is an archetypal image of and guiding principle for a Christian social culture and leadership quality. The capacity for peace results from active work to mediate between opposites, to let our own activity be guided by the needs of our surroundings.

Counter-images of a leadership practice that respects human dignity

The French revolutionary politician Robespierre stands as a historic example of a thinking which, in pursuance of the ideals of liberty, equality and fraternity, lost touch with the heart. Where this occurs, guiding principles and ideals turn into an ideology in which many become emotionally subordinate and dependent on one charismatic personality – in spiritual terms on inspirations from Lucifer.

Ahrimanic inspirations are at work where this ideological orientation is compounded by the will and an external imposition of power and authority.[59] Various types of totalitarian systems and authoritarian styles of leadership arise. These are characterised by the use of both ideological and practical constraints as instruments of power, including financial shortages in order to achieve certain goals.

Common to both luciferically and ahrimanically inspired social cultures is the greater or lesser restriction on the individual freedom to think, freedom of expression and freedom of action, along with heartless and inhumane elements in ways of behaving and reaching agreement.

We can protect ourselves against the fascination of Lucifer through love for real life: "Those who take spiritual science seriously are not concerned with battling about different professions of faith but instead they wish to pursue serious work in all areas of practical life."[60] We can protect ourselves against the dangers of Ahriman by respecting each person's individual freedom: "The individual should first separate themselves from their associations and connections so that the social element could be realised out of the individuality."[61]

Organising our own modes and structures of work in as conscious and healing a way as possible for social life is therefore the core social task of the Medical Section and the professional associations and institutions affiliated with it.

The working principles set out by Rudolf Steiner

The principle of heartfelt warmth: How can the Anthroposophical Society, the School, the anthroposophical movement and the public work together constructively? As a guiding principle, Steiner drew the sketch illustrated above (see page 30) on the blackboard. He described as follows the working attitude necessary for realising this guiding principle: "It is very important that we acquire the outlook that it is not as if we had a right to give people something other than what they want, as if we had the right to place ourselves above the people to whom we wish to give something. We must rid ourselves of the habit of assuming a didactic or campaigning stance, so that we can really make insight and understanding the basic element of life in the Anthroposophical Society."[62]

A "culture of heartfelt warmth" lives from insight into the needs and necessities of our surroundings, in other words people, and what the matter in hand needs. It creates structures and institutions to satisfy these needs and necessities in the best possible way. Just as the heart can only beat when it perceives the state of life of the organism and the peripheral circulation stirs, the contribution of the individual to the whole also can only integrate itself in a healthy way when it is needed and guided by the perception of the whole it wishes to serve.

Igniting our own power of initiative on the needs of our social environment and becoming creative for it is at the same time the schooling path of selflessness which is so necessary. Because no one can be selfless unless they have a "self". Developing the latter so powerfully that it can abstain from looking at itself – that is our cultural task. The greatest freedom which can be achieved is precisely the freedom from ourselves, being able to abstain from looking at ourselves and turning towards the other without thereby being "diminished", losing something or missing something.[63]

Thus, Steiner allows the forms of collaboration he proposes to interpenetrate each other in his structural sketch.

Thus the vertical element stands at the centre – as a fundamental orientation for each individual who feels an obligation towards one or several Section impulses in their work. It stands for the anthropos, the upright human being, who by virtue of their insight can turn their heartfelt warmth right and left towards the various work contexts of anthroposophical life, but also upwards towards inspiration from the spiritual world and downwards by standing within life with all the demands of the everyday personal, professional and social world of humanity.

The principle of individuality: Rudolf Steiner placed the statutes and the discussion about the statutes of the Anthroposophical Society on a democratic and republican footing:[64] Each member has the right to set themselves goals either in a location or with regard to a subject field, establish a work environment and organise themselves with independent statutes. The only condition is that these individual goals and statutes should not contradict those of the Anthroposophical Society. Here the full scope of the principle of individuality applies.

The principle of fraternity in spiritual community: The School of Spiritual Science is structured in accordance with the principle of spiritual fraternity: the spiritual bond is formed by the three conditions (see page 31) which regulate the various forms of collaboration.

The principle of representation and service: The anthroposophical medical movement – like the other sections – is designed to be community for the provision of services. The School of Spiritual Science should make the findings of anthroposophical spiritual research productive for "fraternity in human coexistence", "for moral and religious life, and for artistic and cultural life in general".[65]

Central to this is the concern of Rosicrucian schooling: "An action performed from goodness of heart is one in which the person who performs it does not pursue their own interest but that of their fellow human beings. And such an action can be called morally good."[66] "And at all times complete harmony must prevail between external life and initiation."[67] "Their instruction [from good spiritual teachers] leads either to good results or otherwise to nothing at all."[68] "They are merely concerned with the development and liberation of all beings who are both human beings and the companions of human beings."[69]

And in building on the impulses of the Rosicrucians, the Templar Order and Goethe's relationship with the continuing activity of the spirit of these communities, Steiner formulated a kind of guiding principle for the current cultural epoch: "And in human beings who were again and again inspired from this side, in whom there continued to live what was to be killed off by burning the Knights Templar, in human beings who were inspired by this, there continued to live the supreme ideal that what creates strife and discord in human beings must be replaced by what can bring goodness to earth in the way that it can be imagined – this goodness – below the symbol of the cross in connection with the roses."[70]

Principle of flexible structures: The nature of the activity of the heart is rhythmical continuity. It is also – the healthier the heart is – the ability to adapt with the greatest possible elasticity to the requirements of the organism. Hence Rudolf Steiner demands of organisations – particularly in the context of his social science lectures – that they should not only be created but that they should also dissolve again in a way that serves life best. Money, too, should be allowed to age and not continue to increase "forever".

Thus it is true of the anthroposophic medical movement, for example, with all its different work situations, that it keeps having to adapt to growing demands and to withdraw from where it is not necessarily needed. Where a hierarchy of skills is needed, this will be set up. Where all are needed and should be involved, democratic arrangements will be made. In other respects tasks can be mandated for a defined period (see page 67), new bodies can be created, and structures that are no longer needed can be dissolved.

All the modes of work developed or suggested by Rudolf Steiner were flexible answers to questions or needs of the time. This principle assures the developmental openness with which both possible stagnation and chaotic phenomena of upheaval and dissolution can be countered in the social sphere.

Centre and periphery of the Medical Section – the crucial change of perspective

When Rudolf Steiner died in 1925, many members and friends experienced how the working community he founded at the Christmas Conference unites the living and the dead. Today many people sense this, too. Steiner's departure from the physical world did not end his collaboration in this community but continued it in a spiritual way. Thus his statement about anthroposophy as the "science of the Grail" and the ideal of community building "in the service of the Grail" became a certainty for many after his death.[71] For the Grail community, in the historical image of the Swan Knights which belong to it, includes the dead who are connected with the living.

During the administrative interregnum after Ita Wegman was dismissed in 1935 by a resolution of the members of the Anthroposophical Society, and until this resolution was formally cancelled and revoked at the first annual general meeting of the Anthroposophical Society after the Second World War in 1948, next to nothing was accomplished at the Goetheanum in the field of medicine.

But Wegman – released from her duties on the executive council of the Anthroposophical Society – undauntedly continued to develop her initiatives and activities for Anthroposophic Medicine in the sphere of her mandate in the School of Spiritual Science. This, as set out in the founding statutes of the Anthroposophical Society, was not affected by members' resolutions. She remained true to her appointment through Rudolf Steiner as the head of the Medical Section for the whole of her life.[72]

Her work continued without interruption and had an international impact. Through Ita Wegman's work the "spiritually peripheral" aspect became all the stronger alongside the physical Goetheanum and the people working there. After Steiner's death, an inversion had occurred. Manfred Klett, for many years the head of the Section for Agriculture, repeatedly experienced this inversion clearly in the course of his work and recorded his experiences in this respect and the insights he obtained in a small publication.[73]

Specifically this means that Rudolf Steiner can work to inspire people everywhere from out of the spiritual world wherever they seek to confer spiritually with him. The more that the Goetheanum was overshadowed after Steiner's death by infighting and crises, and the "heart" was less of an impulse-giving centre and rather more of a diseased organ, the more powerfully centres of anthroposophical activity developed in the periphery. The stronger the efforts at the periphery also became to do something to heal the ailing centre in order after Steiner's death to work in a healing way within the Anthroposophical Society in view of the leadership struggles and divisive tendencies. Particularly outstanding examples of this were the initiatives of Karl König, Willem Zeylmans van Emmichoven, Jörgen Smit and Clara Kreutzer.

It was precisely this in itself tragic historical phase in the development of the Anthroposophical Society, the School of Spiritual Science and the anthroposophic medical movement which – if looked at positively – offered a sign of the health and flexibility of the social culture established by Steiner. The latter facilitates not only a constructive development of striking synergy but also the capacity to survive social turbulence and injuries without the whole organism collapsing as a consequence. That the anthroposophical movement lives and its peripheral circulation can largely compensate even for periodic heart insufficiency in the form of a split or weak leadership was and is a magnificent psycho-social experience of the global anthroposophical community.

The School collegium today – its appointment and dismissal practice

The idea of the School collegium has been in existence since it was founded at the Christmas Conference in 1923/24. As the college of section leaders, it was intended to be the "directorate"[74] of an "autonomous institution", functioning as the "natural soul" of the Anthroposophical Society and advising the latter's executive council in all matters concerning the School.[75] In reality, however, it was first introduced to the public as being in existence at the Michaelmas conference in 2000 by the then chairman of the General Anthroposophical Society, Manfred Schmidt-Brabant. But it has still not been properly put into practice. The ensouled collaboration with the Anthroposophical Society and the establishment of the legal basis of the School as an "autonomous institution" are well on the way but still not full reality. An important developmental step in this direction was the Goetheanum leadership process which was enabled in 2012 and 2013 with the help of the management consultant and friend of the Goetheanum, Dr Friedrich Glasl.[76] The collegium of the School and the executive council of the General Anthroposophical Society now together form a new organ: the Goetheanum leadership. The Goetheanum leadership works together on specific subjects even if there are not yet regular meetings of this leadership organ.

The appointment process for a new section leader range from the establishment of an appointing commission, through a direct appointment following suggestions from the previous section head, to proposals received from the professional movements themselves or their responsible representatives and committees. A decision on appointment is then taken by the Goetheanum leadership.

The task of the Section head, like that of an executive council member of the Anthroposophical Society, was regarded by Steiner originally as a lifelong commitment. Currently at the Goetheanum the time in office is seen as having to be individually determined and reviewed from time to time – although, as before, a degree of commitment and responsibility is expected which equates with the lifelong task. The crucial aspect for continuing the work, or a reason to relinquish it, is whether or not it continues to be productive.

Funding modes within the School as illustrated by the Medical Section

Up to 2001, financing the sections – and thus also the Medical Section – was a pragmatic issue. The Medical Section largely financed itself through its daily work. Conferences, lecturing and donations brought in sufficient income to take care of staff salaries and office supplies, as well as any necessary purchases. This was, however, contingent on heated premises being provided and the Anthroposophical Society also guaranteeing any deficits. Conversely the Medical Section regularly transferred any existing annual surpluses to the Anthroposophical Society.

But in 2001 a great deal changed. Three new members of the executive council arrived: Sergej Prokofieff, Bodo von Plato and Cornelius Pietzner (as treasurer). The financial contribution from the Anthroposophical Society to the Medical Section was limited to 150,000 Swiss francs per year – including all human resources costs for the section head and staff. In other words, funding now comprised an average of ten percent of the Medical Section's overall annual budget.

With its larger administration, the section required bigger premises and more staff and moved out of its two rooms in the Goetheanum into its own building. One office remained at the Goetheanum to maintain the section's presence there. Ruth Andrea – previously the manager as well as assistant to the section head – decided to take on the management of the Dora Gutbrod School of Speech. It did not prove possible, however, in the remaining six months before she left to find a capable successor, let alone induct them into the work.

Given this situation, there was good reason to close the section temporarily "for alterations" or to put the leadership post up for discussion. But neither happened for reasons of continuity. The inevitable administrative turbulence that arose as a consequence was not easy to manage. The initially overwhelmed staff members ensured continuity of work to some extent, but were no longer able to relieve the section head for other tasks. During subsequent years, however, it was possible for the Medical Section to make the transition from its pioneering phase (two to four staff in a small space) to team-oriented organisational and integrative development.

Thus today, now that the working conditions have significantly been consolidated, it has become one of the most urgent tasks also to work on coherent financing for the increased administration of the Medical Section as well as its fields of activity and their coordinating management function in the IKAM collegium (see page 57 ff.)

The Medical Section currently receives its financial resources from three sources:

- Grants from the Anthroposophical Society and contributions from the co-workers of the Medical Section.
- Contributions on own account from events, lectures and congresses.
- Project financing, unallocated donations

Income and expenditure are published annually in the financial report which is part of the annual report of the Medical Section. The proper use of funds in line with the statutes is guaranteed through audit by an auditor. The IKAM coordination fields are financed by the relevant field wherever this is possible. This is done through donations, membership contributions, project funding or income from events. Accountability for the use of funding is rendered to the respective coordination field. If a coordination field cannot fund itself, the management of the Medical Section attempts to fill the funding gap through fundraising or from its own sources.

From the Filder Group to the International Coordination of Anthroposophic Medicine/ IKAM

Michaela Glöckler

The need to step up the work and coordinate the various branches and areas of work of the anthroposophic medical movement became increasingly evident not only at the Goetheanum but also internationally, especially in Germany. The coordination work among the representatives of the anthroposophic medical movement, which had existed since the founding of the Filder Group by Jürgen Schürholz in 1986, continued to develop. The work of this large working group of physicians', manufacturers' and consumers' representatives, which met twice a year at the Filder Clinic as the "Filder Group" up to the turn of the century, led to the formation of the International Coordination of Anthroposophic Medicine (IKAM).

Holger Schüle, the prematurely deceased then managing director of Wala, crucially carried forward this new social development at the turn of the century. He was involved in planning ESAM, the "European Coordination of Anthroposophic Medicine" he was intending to establish, which was the crucial intermediate stage between the Filder Group and IKAM. As a young entrepreneur, it was immediately clear to him that the anthroposophic medical movement as a whole needed a transparent structure and a leadership perspective. After his death, it was initially very difficult to continue the process of further structural development that had been started with such commitment, especially since the previously mentioned additional interim stresses were still having an effect on the administration of the Medical Section.

The appointment of IKAM coordinators

The practice for appointing coordinators is analogous to that for appointing section leaders. Rudolf Steiner's guiding statement in the context of the statute discussions during the Christmas Conference applies to this: that ultimately it does not really matter whether someone is elected democratically, appointed by "aristocratic" authority, nominated or chosen by some other method – the important thing is that the candidate should be the right one! This, he says, can be seen from the fact that the work thrives.

In the context of the foundation establishment in 1911, Steiner also used the term "interpreting" for the nomination procedure which he himself used when forming the founding executive council of the General Anthroposophical Society and the School collegium in 1923/24. Here the underlying question is: who is already active in a convincing way in the relevant area and needs to acquire only a few additional skills in order to satisfactorily fulfil the new, more comprehensive task? Who has been overlooked and might be worth considering? And who should receive additional affirmation, for example in a democratic process?

In other words, this is a process which, in line with "moral intuition", should take place out of love for the matter in hand and be inspired by it.[77] If those involved are concerned to ensure that the work thrives, then personal ambitions can more easily be regulated than if they are primarily guided by the rules of democratic and political power. To clarify this, here are a few examples of the appointment of IKAM coordinators:

Rüdiger Grimm was proposed and inducted by his predecessor Johannes Denger – affirmed by the Council for Curative Education and Social Therapy of the time and the section head. What currently goes by the name of the Council for Curative Education and Social Therapy is the result of their years of ongoing social development work. Today Rüdiger Grimm is internationally known and valued as the secretary/coordinator, and basically as the independent head of this field of work. His work as head is also entirely financed out of this field of work, that is to say, out of the movement for special needs education and social therapy.

Rolf Heine was democratically elected by secret, written ballot after discussions in the international initiative group for anthroposophic nursing and then appointed by the section head. Since then, Rolf Heine has been re-elected several times by the democratically organised nursing forum.

Angelika Jaschke came to this function at the request of the section head and by her own initiative. As an executive council member for many years of the German professional association for eurythmy therapy and of the European eurythmy therapy network, she understood the need for international coordination and was prepared to attempt this task. Meanwhile she knows all eurythmy therapists working worldwide by name and has visited almost all countries in which eurythmy therapists are at work. In 2006 she called the first international conference for eurythmy therapy which filled about 90 percent of the large hall of the Goetheanum with eurythmy therapists. The next event in this regard is planned for 2016.

Patrick Sirdey (pharmaceuticals manufacturers) and *Peter Zimmermann* (chairman of the IVAA) were democratically elected umbrella association chairmen and as such legitimate representatives and internationally active coordinators. For Patrick Sirdey there is currently no successor because the AFMUTA association is currently inactive. Thus the Weleda and Wala managements are always welcome as guests and are kept informed about everything happening within the framework of IKAM. Thomas Breitkreuz as successor of Peter Zimmermann has transferred the IKAM mandate to Laura Borghi from the IVAA executive council.

Ad Dekkers and *Henriette Dekkers* were "interpreted" or invited to be coordinators by the section head due to their international presence and the initiatives they have been developing for anthroposophic psychotherapy.

The International Coordination of Anthroposophic Medicines (IMKA) was formed because of the growing need for European and international coordination in relation to maintaining and further developing the range of medicines. *Georg Soldner* took the initiative here, supported by the Executive Council of the IVAA and by the section head. His mandate was officially confirmed nine months later at the next international conference of medical association executive councils at the Goetheanum.

These examples may suffice to give an idea of how IKAM appointments are made in practice.

The structural principles of flexibility, individual initiative, interpretation of skills and capacities, situation-specific appointments and democratic organisational principles can mutually complement each other if it is clear what is needed, what is wanted and if those involved feel themselves to be serving a commonly perceived task.

IKAM's working capacity and efficiency

At the beginning of IKAM's work the question was often raised: is it possible to work efficiently in such a large group? How can everyone have an opportunity to make themselves heard? And to what extent can such a heterogeneous structure, with meetings in changing configurations, make decisions and act?

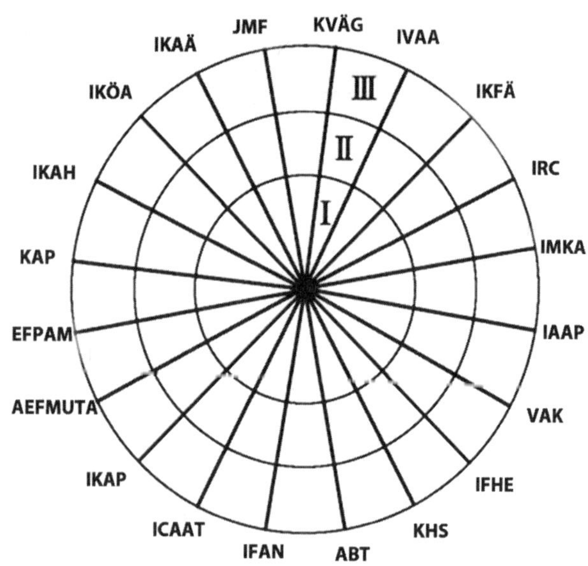

KVÄG	Conference of the Executive Councils of Anthroposophic Medical Associations
IVAA	International Federation of Anthroposophic Medical Associations
IKFÄ	International Coordination of Anthroposophic Specialist Physicians
IRC	International Research Council
IMKA	International Coordination of Anthroposophic Medicines
IAAP	International Coordination of Anthroposophic Pharmacists
VAK	Association of Anthroposophic Clinics
IFHE	International Eurythmy Therapy Grouping
KHS	Council for Curative Education and Social Therapy
ABT	International Coordination of Anthroposophic Body Therapy
IFAN	International Forum for Anthroposophic Nursing
ICAAT	International Coordination of Anthroposophic Art Therapies
IKAP	International Coordination of Age Culture and Elderly Care
AEFMUTA	Association Européenne des Fabricants de Médicaments utilisés en Thérapeutique Anthroposophique
EFPAM	Patient organisations and European Federation of Patients' Associations for Anthroposophic Medicine
KAP	International Coordination of Anthroposophic Psychotherapy
IKAH	International Coordination of Anthroposophic Midwifery
IKÖA	International Coordination of Public Relations
IKAÄ	International Coordination of Anthroposophic Medical Training
JMF	International Young Medics Forum

How this can work is set out in the following chapter. For clarification, the diagram displayed here shows the IKAM organogram in its entirety. The circle as a whole represents the common ground of the anthroposophic medical movement and the Medical Section of the School of Spiritual Science with its worldwide character. Each segment corresponds to a coordination field and its representative.

Other coordination fields are still being developed and are not currently occupied, such as for example drug treatment. At the same time the circle can be extended at any time as new coordination fields arise.

The concentric circles – indicated by Roman numerals in the above diagram – mark the boundaries between the three spheres of the social organism:

1. Research, training and further training – the sphere of intellectual and cultural life and individualism.
2. The legal sphere, professional associations – the sphere of rights and political life, democracy, negotiation and agreements.
3. Economic life, institutions – the sphere of fraternal associative life.

There are meanwhile countries in which the entire anthroposophical medical movement is reflected regionally. Forms of organisation range from tightly organised umbrella associations, such as the Umbrella Association for Anthroposophic Medicine in Germany (DAMiD) to looser network structures, such as those cultivated in the Netherlands and Switzerland.

Why individual representatives and not collegiums to head the individual coordination fields?

As work and also professional demands increase, the question arises as to whether the symmetrical interaction of individual and collegial responsibility favoured by Steiner ought to be changed to primarily collegial work structures. It seems to us that Rudolf Steiner's model – of affirming individual responsibility in a symmetrical and clearly defined way in contrast to collegial structures in organising social relationships – will prove to be ever more relevant in the future.

Why is that so?

- Shared responsibility lacks the binding, "total" commitment to the whole.

- The representatives of 20 work fields can easily and flexibly communicate and work with one another – even with two or three times as many people this become difficult or no longer possible or efficient.
- In undivided responsibility, the inner commitment to the task grows and thus also the associated sense of taking it seriously.
- An individual feels the necessity of collaborating with many others more quickly than a collegium. He or she learns to delegate and to mandate.
- Public representation gains greater transparency and commitment if the contact person is clearly defined without "retreating into the collegium".
- The flexibility of collegial structures is frequently inadequate; furthermore, it can often take a lot of time to reach agreement, etc., which is lost for working.
- If individuals have an overview of a large work area, it is easier for the whole to be aware of itself.
- It is self-evident that an individual who wants to succeed in the task of leading a community can only do so if they are able to lead or are willing to learn to do so: that is to say, the more they are able to distribute as far as possible the pending tasks among the members of the community, give them a mandate and, as necessary, also take care of the financing requirements arising in this connection. Leadership here means being open to the developmental requirement of the community and tying oneself down as little as possible with concrete activities which someone else could do just as well. Because the more actively the individual in the community can contribute to the success of the whole, the more the community can develop in a living way.
- It is also a persuasive image, however, that it takes an individual drop to reflect the whole universe. In collegial responsibility there always arises a mix, difficult for the environment to define, of partial responsibilities, complete, limited or also oppositional (non-)backing of decisions. Since, however, an individual cannot in any case cope alone with an international coordination task, this intrinsically supports the intention of structuring the area of responsibility, developing contacts, forming teams and building networks as required,

which in any case necessitates collaboration within one's own internationally distributed area of responsibility.

- Individual responsibility makes the flexible interaction and collaboration in IKAM with the coordinators from other areas of responsibility possible. The latter can easily and clearly come together to take collegial overall responsibility for the anthroposophic medical movement.[78]
- It is the task of the fifth post-Atlantean cultural epoch to develop the personality, the competence of the I, and the process of learning how the individual can constructively integrate themselves into their social environment. That is to say, it is necessary to practise Rudolf Steiner's "motto of social ethics" quoted at the beginning. It is counterproductive, on the other hand, to claim that there were no longer any "great" personalities and that the work therefore had to be delegated to teams of "minor" personalities. In truth this hides possible concerns that the individual might become too powerful or not be up to the task, the need for social control, or sometimes also jealousy and resentment. We want to confront this and support the power of initiative of the individual person.

Questions and answers about our leadership concept

Rolf Heine

The previous chapters set out the history and development of the Medical Section in the context of Rudolf Steiner's leadership intentions. The reception of the first edition triggered a major discussion process, as already indicated in the foreword. We will now seek to provide some explanations using the most important questions and criticisms. The attentive reader will notice that some things have already been discussed in the previous text. We have, however, deliberately retained the more dialogical form to keep the development of the text transparent in comparison to the first edition.

How can the form of working described here do justice to the developmental conditions of the anthroposophic medical movement?

The anthroposophic medical movement consists of many thousands of people spread over all continents: people in the greatest variety of health profession, sometimes associated in an anthroposophically oriented enterprise, sometimes in professional organisations, anthroposophical branches or independent working groups, sometimes self-employed, sometimes completely on their own without any anthroposophically-minded surroundings.

Ultimately they are united by the heart-felt need for a spirit-filled medicine which respects the human being, inspired by Rudolf Steiner's anthroposophy. This need is founded in a world-spanning community of people in whose heart it is inscribed. This community is the Medical Section of the School of Spiritual Science. Everyone who feels that they belong to it is its member, its co-worker. Here there are three stages, or three levels of intensity of involvement in the Medical Section:

- Involvement in an area of the anthroposophic medical movement.
- Membership of the Anthroposophical Society to study anthroposophy and support the School.
- Membership of the First Class of the School of Spiritual Science for deeper study of Anthroposophic Medicine, the cultivation of the spiritual community and representation of Anthroposophic Medicine in public.

This self-selected form of involvement does not, however, give rise to any rights, merely self-chosen inner or outer obligations.

The Medical Section has a physical centre at the Goetheanum in Dornach. It is represented by its co-workers and the section head. The section head faces the same inner challenges in the esoteric field as every other co-worker of the anthroposophic medical movement worldwide. Professionally it is responsible above all for the administrative services to support Anthroposophic Medicine in the three fields of the social organism: the intellectual and cultural sphere, the sphere of rights and the economic and social sphere. Rudolf Steiner speaks in this context of ad"ministration" in a good sense. It collects, collates and coordinates initiatives in the field of Anthroposophic Medicine worldwide. Exoteric and esoteric training, research and practice belong into its field of awareness and activity as do general cultural and societal developments.

But these self-chosen tasks do not give rise to any rights for the section head either. The section head cannot by virtue of their office or any financial budget dispose over anything but can only make suggestions and facilitate. Everything they do on their own initiative can only become socially effective if there is a resonance in the anthroposophic medical movement. It can only take effect through insight and enthusiasm. Or, as set out above: the heart can only beat healthily if the peripheral circulation is active and everyone does what is needed.[79]

A threefold Christian structural principle can be identified in such a "leadership pattern of deliberate powerlessness":

- Any individual who wishes to set up an initiative in the world needs to combine with other people.
- The community which thus arises around a given task freely agrees the rules of its collaboration.
- Then people support one another in a fraternal way and thus contribute together to the success of the project.

But this threefold ideal is open to attack and at risk in many different ways, as the diagram below shows. Because already existing working communities such as umbrella associations, professional organisations or enterprises give rise to different organisational impulses than those from an individual who commits themselves in freedom to a task. They act as corporate bodies, not as single, individual people. In order to set up initiatives in the world, they commission people with tasks and assign them competences. Organisations and companies delegate and assign mandates.

In contrast, the individual sponsor of an initiative is only responsible to themselves. The bearer of a mandate serves their organisation. But both require the capacity of social awareness, the willingness to compromise and the technical skills to realise the task to be performed – if the latter is to succeed and have a beneficial effect. Individual sponsors of an initiative are open to attack, just as organisations are, and subject to danger from two sides, as the diagram on the next page shows.

These two social organisational principles, the principle of individuality and the organ principle meet in the Medical Section. They are dependent on one another and can supplement one another constructively:

Businesses, institutions and associations adopt important functions arising from the "organ principle" within their respective national or international legal frameworks. They contribute to defining and structuring the public life of Anthroposophic Medicine. Through their activity it has a presence in cultural and economic life. Through the "principle of individuality" of single people and their collaboration with others on their own responsibility and with their own intent inside and outside institutions, beneficial ideas and human warmth come to expres-

Ahrimanic impulses such as abuse of office and power	**Principle of individuality** Self-commitment based on free initiative	Luciferic impulses such as personal vanity and ambition
Social consequences:	***Social consequences:***	***Social consequences:***
Cliqueiness	Voluntary association	Esoteric group
Pedantry	Voluntary agreements	Arbitrariness
Money for influence	Fraternal collaboration	Cronyism
Efficiency is when I can utilise the skills of people and financial resources to optimise the growth in my power.	"The healthy social life is found when in the mirror of each human soul the whole community finds its reflection and when in the community the virtue of each one is living." Rudolf Steiner	The greatest benefit to my "image" is when others admire me for my skills and I can act on the "strength" of my position.
Force of necessity "without alternatives"	Relevant skills	Amateurishness
Tactical compromise	Ability to compromise	Rotten compromise
Abuse of office/power	Mandate	Corruption
	Service obligation Assignment	
	Organ principle	

sion. Organisations and businesses are dependent on such a spiritual inflow of developing ideas just as an individual initiative – to be successful – has to connect with existing communities and services.

Within the IKAM structure the organisation principle and the principle of individuality penetrate one another both in the composition of the coordination centres and in daily working practice. An example of a coordination centre which is represented by the delegate from an umbrella association is the International Federation of Anthroposophic Medical Associations (IVAA).

Examples of individual representations are the profession coordinators who represent a professional group but do not appear as the representatives of a professional association. But all IKAM decisions of relevance for the professional group are nevertheless communicated within the professional group and agreed as relevant.

All IKAM coordinators may and should introduce initiatives to the collegium and develop them further jointly or independently. Only communication, consultation and agreements with the relevant responsible and sponsoring organisations of the movement will ensure the success and sustainability of initiatives.

The management and leadership instruments put into practice by Rudolf Steiner combined the principle of individuality and organ principle in the respective factual context in a coherent way. Thus he used democratic means where existing communities, offices and tasks required the consent of many – ideally of everyone. In establishing new initiatives he "interpreted" (sought) co-workers on the basis of their skills and "suitability". In collegiums matters which concern the whole were discussed on a republican basis and decisions were taken as far as possible unanimously.

Why is the Christmas Conference of 1923 always cited when issues of working structures which are appropriate for our time arise? Have more modern organisational forms and methods not been developed in the meantime, not least in anthroposophical social research?

Just because something was good in the past does not mean that it is still valid as such today. But we are interested in the modes of working which Rudolf Steiner himself used in leading the Anthroposophical Society and to which Ita Wegman committed herself as section head from 1923 to her death in 1943.

These modes of working which Rudolf Steiner used are our guiding star, ideal and path of schooling. They are revealed here as the inner guidance for the IKAM co-workers. Why is that so? Because the Goetheanum and with it the Medical Section are Rudolf Steiner's work, his last – social – edifice. We think that he and his intentions should be facilitated at the Goetheanum and not a social researcher of the present. After all, the latter has the whole world at their disposal.

Furthermore, the Christmas Conference with its design for the social organisation of the anthroposophical movement as a whole was, in the words of Rudolf Steiner, an impulse of the future. It was not oriented towards the next ten, fifty or hundred years. We see it as our task to discover this future aspect and to create and put into practice the required working instruments.

Of course we can demand binding consent for socially creative work of this kind from no one but ourselves. Rudolf Steiner thus repeatedly referred to the "free contractual relationship" of mutual acceptance and the will to collaborate.

What are IKAM's tasks?
What is a leadership organ and why is it required? Who or what is to be led?

The anthroposophic medical movement is a world-wide movement which is represented in a good 80 countries on all continents. It can easily be seen that an international coordination is useful, necessary and efficient for developing a common awareness of the numerous regional and national initiatives, communicating them to each other, recognising developments of contemporary and cultural relevance, protecting Anthroposophic Medicine against threats and maintaining a consonant appearance.

The question nevertheless arises as to whether the spiritual source of Anthroposophic Medicine should be maintained from the centre or whether such care is not the task of each individual person? Are we capable at all of doing justice to Rudolf Steiner's intentions with regard to an esoteric way of working in the social sphere? Or must such an attempt inevitably end up in sectarian, illusory or demandingly exclusive forms?

We are aware of this risk! But we see it above all when administration and esotericism are separated from or played off against one another. Because such a division would reduce administration and management to bureaucratic activities. The spirit would be at risk of turning into "doctrine" or it would only be cultivated any longer in groups divorced from life. If, in contrast, a Christian spirit rules also in the administration and a Christ-inspired moral technique in everyday activities determines the relationship with esoteric truths, then we can counter the pathologies just mentioned.

That is why the attempt is made here to describe spiritual leadership – spiritual administration – spiritual coordination. The sources for this are Rudolf Steiner's management and leadership principles. It remains a risk as to whether we can sufficiently understand and live these principles. But it seems irresponsible to us not at least to try.

Management in Steiner's view is, to begin with, the way that each person manages and leads themselves. Furthermore, it involves being the conduit for ideals, impulses and insights which are accessible to everyone involved in the work – not just to the person who leads or coordinates it. They specifically cannot rely on "special" knowledge because their "power" lies in the mandate to "act on" behalf of the community and not to "instruct" it. In the twelfth lecture of the Curative Education Course Rudolf Steiner explains with the greatest commitment this crucial difference in having such "authority – not in instructing but in acting" with reference to the leadership questions.[80]

In a third step, management is a service for the community. It is not the stronger or more intelligent person imposing their will on the weaker one, the wealthier person on the poorer one or the charismatic person on the more unobtrusive one.

How is agreement reached within IKAM? Are there conflicts of interest among IKAM representatives who belong to an institution / organisation? How are such conflicts of interest handled?

Agreements in IKAM are reached unanimously after proper discussion, including with the help of experts as necessary.

Decisions vetoed by any individual are not admissible. In order to allow for a majority decision to be tolerated, the reasons for rejecting the majority decision are documented and the person objecting is released from their responsibility for the decision at their request. If the veto is maintained, individual co-workers alone or jointly may still take action proactively even if the IKAM collegium as a whole does not wish to become part of their initiative. They are then acting on the basis of their individual competence but not as IKAM representatives.

We are of the opinion that the striving for power and enforcement of individual interests against material objections from others can just as much put the movement as a whole at risk as the paralysis of initiatives through enforced unanimity.

Conflicts of interest can and must exist. When they are

revealed, it becomes evident why a certain view or attitude is held and much can be learnt from that. As the perspectives from which the respective IKAM representatives are speaking is known, and it is possible to have a sense of the degree to which they are capable of placing their own "institutional interests" in the context of the whole, conflicts of interest do not of necessity need to have a negative impact on decisions.

What is the position of specific bodies, for example umbrella organisations or medical associations, within the Medical Section?
What legitimacy do decisions of a body (IKAM) which itself is not democratically legitimised have for itself?

Umbrella organisations, professional associations and other bodies such as enterprises or associations are necessary for acting within the respective national or international legal frameworks. They are part of the anthroposophic medical movement and in their field also assume central tasks on behalf of the whole. They are therefore included to the optimum degree in the leadership of the Medical Section, either as a direct coordination field within IKAM or as represented by a coordinator. But there should be no "party whip" for the IKAM representative from an organisation. On the contrary, they must ask themselves in any decision-making process what they themselves can support and – as described above – abstain or put in a veto as appropriate.

Decisions taken in IKAM cannot therefore be directed against individual parts of the anthroposophic medical movement since it is the persons in positions of responsibility who work in IKAM with the overall context in mind beyond their own specialist interests. No matter whether IKAM decisions are welcomed or rejected, it is anyway the case that they can only be implemented to the extent that those who understand themselves to be co-workers of the Medical Section want to implement them. Where this does not happen, something else or nothing at all comes about.

The same applies to the recognition and legitimisation essentially required by IKAM from the movement as a whole or its co-workers, institutions and organisations. IKAM is either wanted and thus becomes effective or not and is thus weakened. The concept of freedom and initiative is its strength and weakness. IKAM is strengthened if, for example, democratically elected organisations recognise it by their own democratic rules. This can happen in that the connection with the Medical Section is included in their statutes, members are informed about its activities and/or the work of the Medical Section is financially supported.

To what extent has the threefold structure of the social organism proposed by Rudolf Steiner been taken into account in the responsibility structure of the Medical Section?

To begin with, the threefold structure of the social organism is a fact like the threefold structure of the human organism. It is not a social utopia which will only be achieved a long way into the future. Just like in the human organism, we can diagnose the disorders and trends in the social organism against the background of social threefolding. The Medical Section – as co-organiser of the School of Spiritual Science as a place for the study of medical subjects and as a community of people working in the spirit of Anthroposophic Medicine – is an organ of the cultural and intellectual life. Hence the primacy of the principle of freedom and individuality in every type of structure is rigorously set out in this publication.

This principle of freedom also characterises the rights sphere of the Medical Section in the sense of its self-governance structures. In the context of a valid, reliable framework of agreements, these structures are presented, for example, for IKAM in this publication. Every co-worker of the Medical Section has the possibility of introducing their initiative on an equal basis. There is no instance that can impede an initiative. There are transparent advisory bodies and leadership structures. The leadership is given the powers it needs to fulfil its tasks. Coordination and integration determine its mode of working. In order to execute legal transactions with third parties, it uses bodies such as associations or foundations. In the international legal sphere it is trying to obtain recognition as an NGO.

The Medical Section participates in the economic life as the provider of various services. It organises conferences and coordinates, publishes, facilitates and undertakes research. In doing so, it never acts in competition with other initiatives but rather makes its expertise and infrastructure available to them. This principle of economic activity means that it is also dependent on generous financial contributions from the anthroposophic medical movement and from other beneficiaries of its services.

The Medical Section and its leadership has an existential interest in the medical and ethical developments in medicine, but also in the legal and political as well as the economic framework conditions within which individuals or facilities of the anthroposophic medical movement act nationally and internationally. This interest and commitment is founded in the remit and statutes of the Christmas Conference. Hence representatives both from the professional specialist groups and from politically active fields (e.g. AnthroMed or the IVAA) or representatives from economic enterprises (e.g. pharmaceutical manufacturers, clinic association) sit in the IKAM collegium and their fields of work are correspondingly shown in the organogram.[81]

What is the position of esoteric working communities such as the First Class of the School of Spiritual Science (Michael School) or the Raphael Group within the Medical Section?

Rudolf Steiner established numerous ways of working esoterically. These range from the personal teacher-pupil relationship, for example with Marie Steiner and Ita Wegman, through to the esoteric schools before the First World War, the foundation of the School of Spiritual Science as part of the Christmas Conference, the help in founding the Christian Community and the Esoteric Youth Circle (Jugendkreis) or the institution of the Raphael Group (see page 207 ff.), to name but the most well-known.

Rudolf Steiner saw his role in their establishment as being a facilitator between the spiritual world and the enquiring people, not as their initiator. The success or failure of these jointly founded initiatives was and is dependent on the possibilities of the people involved and the response which the deeds of these people receive from the spiritual world. As a facilitator, Rudolf Steiner placed himself directly and selflessly in the developmental stream of the communities founded with his involvement with all the karmic consequences this entailed.

Esoteric communities exist because of the inner commitment and spiritual questions which led to their foundation. They make no claim to power and influence. Thus a member of the First Class of the School of Spiritual Science does not possess any outer or inner privileges over any other person. The self-imposed obligation of Class members to meditate on the basis of spiritual science, to "maintain association" and to represent the spirit of anthroposophy merely entails hard work and effort from a social perspective – in no way, however, is it an entitlement to recognition, power of preferment.

Esoteric communities formed within anthroposophy go back to the supersensory Michael School which was founded in the fifteenth century and which is the source out of which anthroposophy is inspired.[82] Joining an esoteric working context happens on initiative of the seeker or on personal invitation.

Ultimately all therapeutic specialisations (professional groups and specialist disciplines) within Anthroposophic Medicine have sought and developed methods of esoteric deepening of life. These are cultivated in free working relationships, free agreements on common meditative practice, meetings of the School of Spiritual Science or specialist conferences. Every specialisation and deepening, each time that knowledge grows or another skill is acquired, poses the risk that we rank ourselves or our peer group above or below, in front or behind others. Such social position fixing disguises the true and real karmic relationships between individual people and their actual tasks both within the community and between the various groupings. In any event, a Christian mystery medicine will only succeed if we develop the ability to make our contribution individually in awareness of the whole or with our work community or institution.

Without love and humour the paths remain hidden by means of which spiritual streams infuse and supplement one another.

Responsibility structures and working instruments of the Medical Section – an overview

The Medical Section at the Goetheanum is a department of the School of Spiritual Science set up by Rudolf Steiner in 1923/24. Its task is to work on the "medical system of anthroposophy" through research into and the dissemination and further development of anthroposophic medicine and the art of healing.

As a working community active throughout the world, the co-workers of the Medical Section require a form of organisation which is compatible both with the conditions of life of a free spiritual life and which is suitable for accommodating "the initiation principle among the civilisational principles". That is, it requires responsibility structures which are based both on each individual's capacity for initiative – a free spiritual life – and yet take account of the diversity of national and regional needs and developments, as well as meeting the needs of evolved work and legal forms on a local and international level. The way in which this has developed and proved itself from the mid-1990s to the present day will be set out below.

1. Collaboration within the Medical Section

There is no formal membership of the Medical Section. Everyone can feel that they belong to it who collaborates on Medical Section tasks and for whom regard of the following conditions is a matter close to their heart:

- General and subject-specific study of anthroposophy alongside continuing professional development (path of knowledge and self-training).
- Participation in working groups and conferences in order to cultivate dialog and collaboration with other Medical Section co-workers (social competence, community building).
- Realisation of Anthroposophic Medicine by serving patients in a professional way and with a sense of responsibility (attitude to life, representation).

2. Areas of work

Like all sections of the School of Spiritual Science, the Medical Section is also active in three areas of work:

- The area of work of institutions and initiatives of the anthroposophic medical movement,
- The area of work of the Anthroposophical Society with its branches and working groups in the field of medicine and the art of healing,
- The purely meditative area of work of the First Class of the School of Spiritual Science.

3. Modes of work of the Medical Section

Spiritual responsibility: The modes of work described here are founded on the conviction that thoughts, feelings and motives for action are not just the expression of an attitude to life but embody a spiritual reality. This gives rise to an individual awareness not just of actions that unfold in the physical world, but also of being responsible for our own thoughts and attitudes.

Initiative principle: The source and starting point for all activities within Anthroposophic Medicine is the personal initiative of individual people. Initiatives for work with patients, multiprofessional and interdisciplinary collaboration, involvement in the development of legal relationships as well as for research and training arise from a free decision and not from statutes or programmes. Thus the foremost task of all leadership organs of the Medical Section is to accompany, support and advise on initiatives.

Individual development: Rudolf Steiner designed the School's sections as places of ongoing development through study, inner schooling and professional collaboration. Many training centres and further training courses, working groups and conferences at the Goetheanum and elsewhere in the world meet this task.

Spiritual scientific research: Spiritual scientific research is founded on the individual path of schooling, the stages of which Rudolf Steiner characterised in detail (GA 10 and 13). The core tasks of all co-workers of the Medical Section include metamorphosing this path into the medical domain and relating it to modern academic research methods or making it generally productive for the medical system.

Remaining in dialogue with one another and maintaining association: In our present cultural epoch, in which each individual must focus on his or her personal developmental needs, it is absolutely indispensable to have a reliable association between people based on trust. Here the Medical Section has the task of fostering dialog among and between the specialist competencies and spiritual qualities of the different medical professions and uniting them in a common whole; for the benefit both of patients and the individual therapist.

Spiritual community building: The Medical Section aims to engage with the talents and weaknesses of its co-workers in a way that supports the individual development of each person so that in give and take a shared, brotherly-sisterly awareness of the community and the needs of the world, which the community serves, can arise.

Representation: Each co-worker of the Medical Section contributes to the development and profile of Anthroposophic Medicine through their actions, feeling and thinking, both in their personal life and in their professional practice. Supporting one another to make individual and social representation relevant in the public sphere is both an aspiration and a challenge.

4. Work organs

The organs of the Medical Section serve to make Anthroposophic Medicine a reality. Each of their co-workers is the starting point from which their idea can be realised. The initiative of individuals is as significant as that which comes from institutions, associations or groups.

Since each of its co-workers is the starting point for potential local action, each single person also functions as an organ within the whole. This gives rise to the following structure:

- The head of the Medical Section.
- The working community of internationally active coordinators of the professional fields and task areas (International Coordination of Anthroposophic Medicine – IKAM).
- The co-workers of the Medical Section worldwide.

4.1. Leadership and understanding of leadership

The understanding of leadership as set out relates to all areas of the Medical Section. In line with this understanding, the section leadership, international coordination (IKAM) and also each single colleague have the task of working integratively and through their own initiative. This also means that the exercise of a leadership task bears fruit to the extent that "managing" and "allowing oneself to be managed", "coordinating" and "being coordinated" are conditional upon each another.

Leadership of a spiritual community requires a structure that values, includes and supports every single co-workers as a source of inspiration and initiative. In this sense the Medical Section is led by individuals who see their task as spiritual service. This means assuming a voluntary commitment, depending on what a situation or task demands. It also follows from this that such an understanding of leadership cannot and does not wish to claim any doctrinal authority founded in an office.

Such an understanding of leadership proves fruitful if the co-workers of the section take the initiative at their respective locations to put Anthroposophic Medicine into practice; and if an awareness of the goal and degree of implementation of such initiatives develops in the organs and leadership structures of the Medical Section. The central leadership tasks follow therefrom:

- Perception of the developmental state of the anthroposophic medical movement.

- Acting as a conduit for spiritual impulses in the sense of altruistically passing on insights, experience and information which could be of help to individuals, groups or institutions.
- Providing impulses, inspiration, integration and coordination for initiatives as required.
- Promoting and maintaining communication and transparency within the anthroposophical medical movement.

The relationship between the centre and periphery as represented in the human organism between the heart and capillaries is also a functional image of and guiding principle for the social organism of the Medical Section.

Tasks of the section head: The head of the Medical Section at the Goetheanum has four task areas:

- They are part of the overall leadership of the Goetheanum.
- They support and coordinate the affairs and developments within the anthroposophic medical movement and their integration into the medicine and art of healing of the present day.
- They develop initiatives wherever this is possible and desired with the aim of supporting the nature, spread and acceptance of Anthroposophic Medicine and establishing it in public life.
- They chair IKAM conferences and appoint coordinators in agreement with the IKAM collegium.

Depending on the requirements of the situation, the head of the Medical Section should observe, be appreciative, integrate, delegate, inspire and give impulses.

Nomination of the head and the Goetheanum leadership: The leader of the Medical Section is appointed by the School collegium following discussion and in binding agreement with IKAM. The IKAM coordinators consult their colleagues in the bodies in which they work and table proposals in the IKAM collegium. IKAM's vote for a nomination is guided by the following criteria:

- The person to be appointed should be capable of understanding and supporting the work and developmental conditions of the professional groups collaborating in the Medical Section.
- The person to be appointed should be able to lead a global organisation administratively and entrepreneurially.
- The person to be appointed should be sufficiently accepted by the co-workers of the Medical Section.
- The person to be appointed should possesses qualities such as charisma, empathy, the capacity to integrate and initiative.

The IKAM collegium is at liberty to choose its selection instruments.

Term in office of head; recall: There is no time limit on the period for which the head can be appointed. If the head can no longer productively fulfil their tasks, they shall be recalled by the collegium of the School of Spiritual Science. A recall request may also be addressed by IKAM to the collegium of the School of Spiritual Science following a unanimous decision.

4.2. *International Coordination of Anthroposophic Medicine (IKAM)*

IKAM is the working group and collegium of the international coordinators of the professional fields and task areas within the Medical Section. The task of IKAM is to monitor and observe jointly the development of the anthroposophic medical movement and to agree and implement initiatives to provide collective help and support. IKAM members each individually bear spiritual and entrepreneurial responsibility for their task area.

The IKAM members are the heart organ of the anthroposophic medical movement and enable the section head to fulfil his or her core task. They table impulses and initiatives arising from the task area or professional field they represent in the IKAM collegium. The justification for doing so arises from insight into the significance, purposefulness or need of the initiatives and impulses concerned for the development of their own task area and/or for the anthropoposophic medical movement as a whole.

Appointment of coordinators: Coordinators of the professional fields and task areas are appointed by the section head in agreement with the representatives of the professional field and task area concerned and with the IKAM collegium.

Term of appointment, recall: Appointments last for as long as the coordinator's work is productive with regard to the professional field and the collaboration with the section head and IKAM. Such productiveness is revealed particularly in the feedback coming from the professional field or task area as well as in the trust that the section head and the IKAM collegium show towards the coordinator.

IKAM develops instruments suitable for regularly ascertaining the feedback to the work of a coordinator within their professional group or their task area, and for deliberating jointly with the section head on continuation of the work they do within IKAM.

The IKAM coordinators: Currently the following professional groups and task areas are represented in IKAM:

- **Professional groups**
  Physicians
  Eurythmy therapy
  Midwives
  Special needs education / social therapy
  Non-medical practitioners
  Body therapy
  Art Therapy
  Nursing
  Pharmacy
  Psychotherapy
  Student work
- **Task areas**
  Facilities for the elderly (Nikodemus Werk)
  Pharmaceutical manufacturers

Research
Work in the School of Spiritual Science
International medical training
(Trainer group in the Medical Section)
Hospital association, AnthroMed
International Coordination of Anthroposophic Medicines (IMKA)
International Federation of Anthroposophic Medical Associations (IVAA)
Public relations work
Patient associations
Legal issues relating to medicines

Working instruments of the International Coordination (IKAM)

IKAM conferences: Serve dialogue, discussion and decision-making on joint initiatives.

Individual initiatives: These are encouraged – they merely require to be communicated and, as necessary, coordinated with colleagues.

Profession coordinators' meetings: The profession coordinators meet as needed, but at least once a year.

Initiative groups: Based on the IKAM rules of procedure, they can be convened and also dissolved again by one or more IKAM members.

Mandate groups: Are commissioned by the section head or by IKAM to fulfil a particular task.

Ad-hoc meetings: Depending on need and situation, ad-hoc meetings can take place or be called between IKAM members at any time, and the results of such meetings are communicated to the IKAM collegium.

The annual conference of the anthroposophic medical movement: Once a year, all the co-workers of the anthroposophic medical movement meet for a conference at the Goetheanum. The annual conference is prepared by the section head and IKAM coordinators. Its purpose is to meet and inspire one another. It is a place in which the anthroposophic medical movement can become aware of itself and, through this self-awareness, draw strength for its task. IKAM coordinators also meet with their networks, forums or work councils and mandate groups; they do so in most instances as part or on the sidelines of the conference itself.

Internal and external communication: IKAM News is an internal communication organ of the IKAM council. It contains short reports from the fields of work of the IKAM coordinators and serves to form and cultivate a common awareness of the worldwide anthroposophic medical movement.

The Newsletter of the Medical Section is regularly sent to the co-workers of the anthroposophic medical movement in at least six languages. It reports on current events, questions, concerns and communication needs; it aims to nurture the spiritual connection between all co-workers worldwide and to be a core instrument of spiritual community building.

The annual report and accounts of the Medical Section contain the report from the section head and the IKAM coordinators – including events at the Goetheanum and cooperations and activities worldwide – as well as the financial statement.

Rules of procedure: IKAM sets its own rules of procedure and can amend these as necessary.

Creative scope for the co-workers of the Medical Section: This arises from personal initiative. Supporting such initiatives is the core task of the head of the Medical Section and IKAM. The election of delegates and other democratic opinion-forming and voting procedures may be used if these are appropriate for the matter of debate. The use of such procedures is determined by the head of the Medical Section and IKAM.

Suitable instruments for ascertaining the degree to which the section head and IKAM are accepted among co-workers of the worldwide medical movement may be deployed as required.

Internal and external legal relationships: As a department in the "School of Spiritual Science, Goetheanum", the Medical Section has the status of a registered private college in the Swiss canton of Solothurn. It awards diplomas and cooperates with many training centres with regard to issues of accreditation and recognition.

The national professional associations are connected with the Medical Section through the profession coordinators. They are subject to the law of their own countries. Together they conclude international and supranational agreements or join together to form international umbrella organisations which support the worldwide, free development of Anthroposophic Medicine and art of healing. Depending on the subject matter, they collaborate in this task with pharmaceutical manufacturers, patient organisations as well as governmental and non-governmental institutions.

Funding principles: The funding of the Medical Section comes from four sources:

- Grants from the Anthroposophical Society.
- Income from services and events for the anthroposophic medical movement.
- Donations from foundations and institutions.
- Contributions from the co-workers of the anthroposophic medical movement to facilitate the networking activities of the IKAM coordinators and projects.

This last flow of funds is of particular importance, reflecting most authentically whether or not the section head and IKAM are fulfilling their tasks as expected by the co-workers of the Medical Section.

4.3. The Medical Section office

The Medical Section runs an office at the Goetheanum in Dornach. Its function is to support the section head in all administrative tasks. The office is the contact point for all co-workers of the Medical Section as well as for cooperation partners and the public. It supports the IKAM coordinators in their tasks.

The fields of work of the International Coordination of Anthroposophic Medicine (IKAM)

and its meditative impulses

The contributions below from the IKAM coordinators of the Medical Section give an insight into the work of the various coordination fields in their day-to-day work for Anthroposophic Medicine.

Conference of the Executive Councils of Anthroposophic Medical Associations

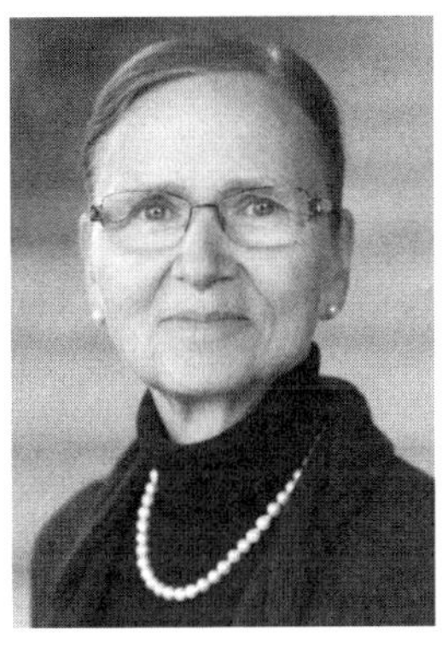

Dr med. Michaela Glöckler
Head of the Medical Section, overall coordination for IKAM
michaela.gloeckler@medsektion-goetheanum.org

Since 1989, the members of the executive councils of all existing anthroposophic medical associations have been invited once a year to meet at the Goetheanum and discuss common questions, tasks and future perspectives. In 2009, the meeting on 15 and 16 September focused on reviewing 20 years of shared work and on the outlook for the future:

- Quo vadis, anthroposophic medical movement?
- Where do we see a need for innovation and scope for new structures and ventures?
- What forms of research, training and further training are there and where do they need to be developed?
- What work instruments and forms does that require? What already exists and only needs to be optimised?
- How is the public relations work that needs to be done positioned?
- What task must be taken up or developed further?
- How can collaboration be structured also with regard to spiritual community building?
- How can the necessary translation work be financially supported so that the most important anthroposophical primary and secondary medical literature is available worldwide?

With regard to these questions there was also discussion as to what has proved itself, what still requires further development and where there is a need for renewal or change.

The Conference of Executive Councils is the central meeting place for representatives from meanwhile 40 medical associations. It instigated the reconstitution of the International Federation of Anthroposophic Medical Associations / IVAA with groups responsible for training, research, the availability of medicines and support for the Vademecum (www.vademecum.org) and the Anthromedics project (www.gaed.de/gaaed/struktur/strukture/anthromedics.html). It is the body in which all internationally important concerns of Anthroposophic Medicine are discussed in their development and which plays a part in reaching a decision on them.

IVAA – International Federation of Anthroposophic Medical Associations – Coordination

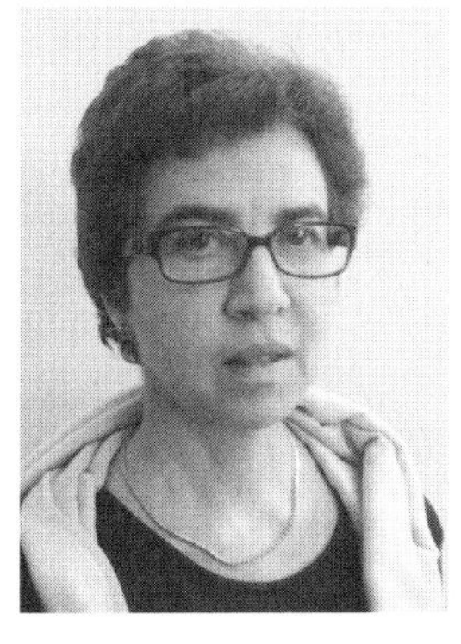

Dr med. Laura Borghi
IVAA council member
Coordinator of the IVAA in IKAM
lauraborghi@medicinaantroposofica.it
www.ivaa.info

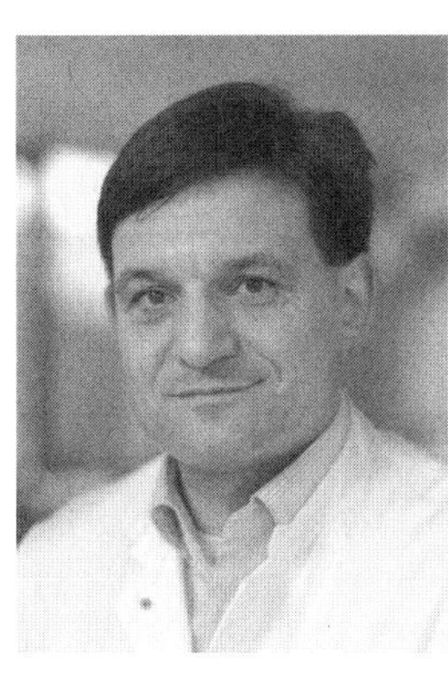

Dr med. Thomas Breitkreuz
President of the IVAA
t.breitkreuz@paracelsus-krankenhaus.de
www.ivaa.info

For how long has the IVAA been in existence? How many member associations does it have? How is it organised?

The IVAA was established in 1992 and is the successor of the IAV (International Anthroposophic Medical Association). It is an association under Swiss law and was registered in the commercial register of the Canton of Solothurn on 7 June 1993 (CH-247.6.000.010). In 2013, the IVAA had medical member associations in 31 countries worldwide, of which 18 were in the EU, with approx. 3200 fully trained anthroposophical physicians in total in 2012. The IVAA delegates represent the national medical associations at the annual general meeting of members (www.ivaa.info). The IVAA is led as per its statutes by an executive council with a maximum of seven members, including a president, vice president and treasurer, which is elected by the annual delegate meeting for a period of three years. Thomas Breitkreuz has been president of the IVAA since September 2013. The head of the Medical Section at the Goetheanum is naturally a member of the IVAA executive council. The IVAA executive council works cooperatively with tasks distributed among its members to undertake on their own responsibility under the leadership and overall coordination of the chairperson. The IVAA is financed from membership fees and project-related funding from foundations with an annual budget of CHF 130,000.

What are the IVAA's tasks?

The task of the IVAA in accordance with its statutes is the worldwide representation of the anthroposophic medical associations in legal and political matters. Regarding its international task, the IVAA currently works primarily within the EU since the recognition of AM and its medicines there is the prerequisite for its spread throughout the rest of the world. It cooperates with other medical associations in complementary medicine in the "CAMDOC Alliance" and beyond that with the relevant CAM associations for patients and non-medical professions in the "EUROCAM" alliance.

The IVAA maintains a permanent presence in Brussels near the EU Parliament and Commission (IVAA EU Liaison Office). With regard to European legislation, the IVAA, looking ahead several years, campaigns for the official recognition and thus brand licensing of AM medicines in the EU. It pursues this goal in close coordination with other AM stakeholders (manufacturers, patients, scientists, pharmacists, therapists), including ESCAMP. ESCAMP is currently working on the scientific prerequisites for the licensing of anthroposophic medicines on the basis of a new concept for verifying their assessment of efficacy within the framework of the overall system of AM. The IVAA is at the same time campaigning for the recognition of CAM in European health policy and is to this end cooperating closely at a European level with the other CAM interest groups; it is also involved in other important initiatives in European health policy.

The IVAA supports the national member associations worldwide with help and advice for legal and political problems in their countries and ensures the feedback of experiences from the individual countries into the international medical community. Outside Europe, the IVAA supports the regional and subject-related collaboration between its member associations.

The IVAA observes its task in the International Coordination of Anthroposophic Medicine IKAM. It represents legally and politically relevant perspectives from the field of Anthroposophic Medicine in the work of IKAM, just as, conversely, the IKAM concerns are conveyed for inclusion in the work of the IVAA executive council and, through the delegates, the anthroposophic medical associations as a whole.

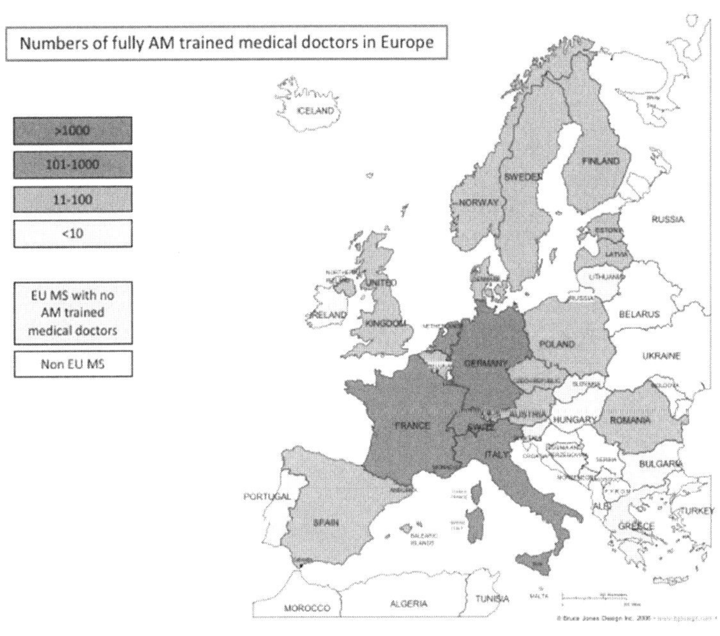

What are the most urgent problems on which the IVAA is working?

At international, European and national level work is taking place appropriately to safeguard the recognition of the overall system of Anthroposophic Medicine and specifically its medical work, as well as the licensing and availability of anthroposophic medicines. The most urgent problem is the absence as yet of recognition for AM medicines in the regulations covering marketing approval for medicines in the EU. A satisfactory solution under national law in this respect has been found in only a few EU member states (incl. Germany) which is not, however, in conformity with the EU system and thus not future-proof. In most other EU member states the current national regulations are unsatisfactory, in some of them AM medicines are even prohibited.

What structures are used to work on these problems?

In its work, the IVAA on the one hand needs to persuade the political decision-makers in the EU institutions (EU Commission, European Parliament and Council) to recognise CAM as an indispensable part of the public health system. This is happening in alliance with the above-mentioned umbrella stakeholders in complementary medicine (CAMDOC, EUROCAM) and at a national level through the corresponding contacts, initiatives and further CAM research (CAMbrella and follow-up projects). On the other hand, the IVAA campaigns for the specific concerns of AM and an appropriate arrangement for AM medicines in the European legislation on human medicine. This work takes place in close collaboration with the other AM organisations. Thus there is close cooperation with ESCAMP, whose scientific work is politically supported by the IVAA and whose proposals for a European medicines regulation are being taken up by the IVAA. There is also an agreement with the patients' association EFPAM, the pharmacists' association IAAP and the manufacturers' association ECHAMP (European Coalition of Homeopathic and Anthroposophic Medicines Producers) as well as with the ELIANT NGO.

Can the principles or references in the work of Rudolf Steiner be used for the political work?

The reference to the threefold order of the social organism is highly relevant for the way the IVAA sees itself and its cooperations. The "fundamental social law" is a lodestar for collaboration in the IVAA executive council.

The IVAA does not contribute to shaping politics as a political lobbying organisation but it works in the awareness of inner guidance arising from "The conditions of esoteric training" in *Knowledge of the Higher Worlds. How is it achieved?* which aim, among other things, to create a balance between the inner and outer world. Here the second condition says: To "feel oneself as a link in the whole of life ... Much is involved in the fulfilment of this condition ... And then it will no longer be an alien thought to consider myself only as a link in the whole of humanity and sharing the responsibility for everything that occurs."

Rudolf Steiner's great appreciation of clarity in legal circumstances and the optimum legal arrangements for work situations is well known.

On 26 December 1923, during the Christmas Conference, he said: "Because if we were to decided today out of some feeling of sympathy no longer to work in the groups except inwardly, something that would no doubt be very nice, were we no longer to care about public opinion, we would see that something would increasingly gain the upper hand in which public opinion takes note of us in a hostile way."[83]

International Coordination of Anthroposophic Medicines / IMKA

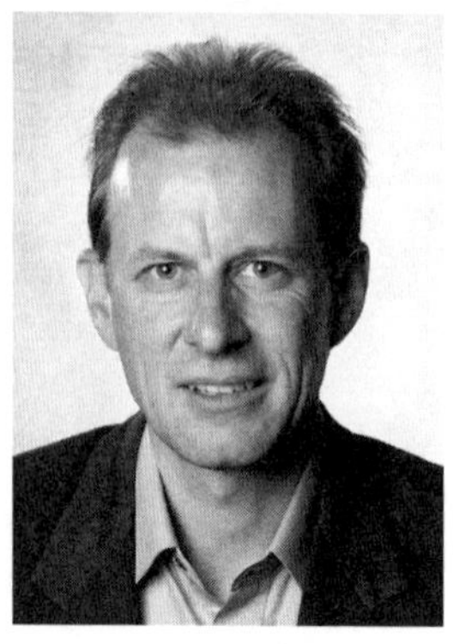

Dr med. Andreas Arendt
International Coordination of Anthroposophic Medicines / IMKA
arendt@bluewin.ch
www.medsektion-goetheanum.org

IMKA's main task is to take up issues and problems arising with regard to anthroposophic medicines across countries, bring them to the attention of the manufacturers or, as necessary, mediate between the needs of the physicians and those of the manufacturers. Andreas Arendt (Switzerland) is IMKA coordinator. He works together with his colleagues and IMKA members Laura Borghi (Italy), Philipp Busche (Germany), Markus Debus (Germany), Reinhard Schwarz (Austria) and Michaela Glöckler (Medical Section, Switzerland). Depending on the task, further persons were included in the group of co-workers.

IMKA's working method

Regular meetings with the manufactures of anthroposophic medicines, as a rule once or twice a year and as required. In these meetings current concerns in the fields of medicinal range, availability, ability to deliver and relating to distribution and research are discussed. Once a year IMKA chairs the joint meeting between the International Conference of Executive Councils of Anthroposophic Medical Associations and the manufacturers. This meeting also offers a platform on which medical representatives from all over the world can personally meet the persons in positions of responsibility at the manufacturers of anthroposophic medicines.

Project: Vademecum of Anthroposophic Medicines

The Vademecum comprises the experience reports on individual medicines from anthroposophic physicians, scrutinised by an international editorial team. The third edition is already available in German. Work on the fourth edition, which will additionally include oncological mistletoe therapy, is currently in progress. The aim is to continue to improve the quality of the Vademecum both through the submission of new experience reports and through critical comments on the already existing and published experiences. Translations of the Vademecum into English, Italian, Spanish and French are in progress or already completed.
www.vademecum.org

International Association of Anthroposophic Pharmacists / IAAP

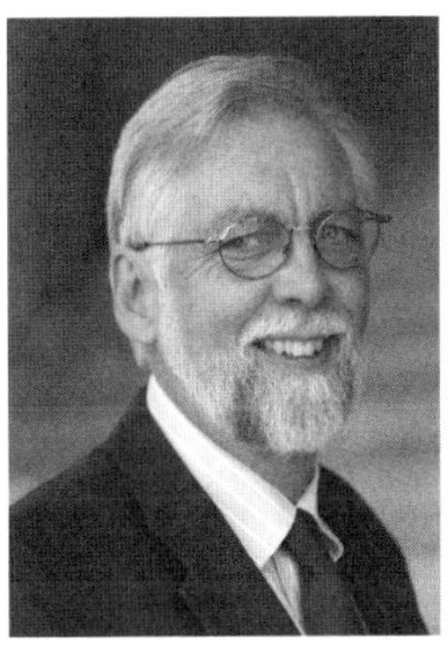

Dr rer. nat. Manfred Kohlhase
IKAM Coordinator for Pharmacy
mail@manfred-kohlhase.de
www.iaap.org.uk

Legal and organisational portrait of the umbrella organisation

The anthroposophically oriented pharmacists as a professional group and their international umbrella association IAAP, established in 2001, joined the Medical Section at the Goetheanum in the same year. The IAAP is an association under Swiss law and today represents seven European national member organisations (in Belgium/Netherlands, Germany, Great Britain, France, Italy, Austria and Switzerland) and a pharmacists' association overseas in Brazil (Farmantropo = Associacao Brasileira de Farmacia Antroposofica). In countries without their own anthroposophic association there is the opportunity to acquire direct IAAP membership as a fellow pharmacist. In Germany (GAPiD) it is meanwhile also possible for pharmaceutical technical assistants to acquire (extraordinary) membership. The establishment of a new association in Japan is in preparation. The executive council consists of representative from the member countries.

In order to create a common, internationally oriented soul and spiritual bond among anthroposophically oriented pharmacists and to reflect the current state of the IAAP's work in personal discussion, the IAAP executive council regularly each year offers an open executive council meeting and a specialist workshop on the APC (Anthroposophic Pharmaceutical Codex) at the annual conference of the Medical Section.

Professional development

Before 2000, there was no common professional awareness or occupational profile among pharmacists who either worked at Abnoba, Helixor, Wala or Weleda (including individual community pharmacists). On suggestion from a colleague at Weleda UK, Manfred Kohlhase set up an initiative group consisting of pharmacists from Weleda and Wala who set themselves the task of drawing up an occupational profile and creating a professional organisation/association with the corresponding statutes. Eleven pharmacists then established the professional association for anthroposophic pharmacists in Germany in 2001. A British association was created in parallel in the same year and initial steps were taken to install the international umbrella association (IAAP). In the following years, further anthroposophic professional associations for pharmacists were founded.

Here the IAAP worked to support and help these newly founded pharmacists' associations in that it drew up guiding statutes and professional guidelines and laid down the conditions for membership of the IAAP.

Groundbreaking was also the development of the international guidelines for the further training of anthroposophic pharmacists, IFEAP = International Further Education in Anthroposophic Pharmacy.

Goals and tasks of the IAAP (services and representation)

The IAAP aims primarily to represent everyone worldwide with an anthroposophical orientation who is working in pharmacy, and wishes to contribute to extending natural scientific pharmacy with spiritual scientific aspects. Here it looks to interdisciplinary collaboration with all colleagues working on an anthroposophical basis in medicine and therapy.

A long-term goal and project has been the publication of the Anthroposophic Pharmaceutical Codex (APC) and its official recognition as a legal pharmacopoeia. Meanwhile two electronic editions are available which are already deemed to be recognised quality documents by the drug licensing authorities in Switzerland, Brazil and Australia and can serve to maintain the market for anthroposophic preparations in those countries. In 2013 the third extended edition also appeared in book form for the first time (see: www.iaap.org.uk).

It also sees a long-term task in the development of internationally valid standards in further and advanced training as well as in the working practices of anthroposophic pharmacists (see IFEAP). Graduates of the advanced training can be certified by the IAAP in accordance with uniform standards and thus obtain the AnthroMed® Pharmacy mark. The long-term objective is a worldwide network of Anthromed® pharmacies which can produce anthroposophic medicines at an extemporaneous level since the staff who make them have passed through a certified advanced training in anthroposophic pharmacy.

It may be possible for the IAAP to contribute in the future to making basic substances listed in the APC available for such pharmacies in countries where there is no supply of anthroposophic medicines.

Financial basis

The work and projects of the IAAP umbrella association are undertaken by the executive council on an honorary basis and have hitherto been financed by membership fees as well as support from the anthroposophical manufacturers. In future, sponsorship money is intended to help reduce the dependence on support from the manufacturers.

A truth-wrought verse – also for pharmacists?

Rudolf Steiner did not give a course specially for pharmacists. But various pharmaceutical aspects, questions and suggestions are contained in the so-called medical courses.[84] In the book *Extending Practical Medicine* (GA 27) in particular, Rudolf Steiner and Ita Wegman devote a separate chapter to the then new typical preparations of Anthroposophic Medicine which have retained their importance to the present day. The first medical course, *Introducing Anthroposophical Medicine* (GA 312), contains a brief treatment of the origin, method and production of homoeopathic medicines and important instructions for mistletoe preparations. In addition, pharmacists will find a wealth of characteristic descriptions of healing substances from all realms of nature – be it minerals, metals, medicinal plants or substances of animal origin – in the whole of Rudolf Steiner's work; in it above all the spiritual and concealed side of this substance world becomes clear and its relationship with human beings and their illnesses is revealed.

The task of the pharmacist has for centuries consisted of acquiring knowledge about natural substances and preparing medicines from them. Such skill in preparing medicines and the profound knowledge of natural substances are largely no longer required in pharmacies and by pharmacists.

Anthroposophic pharmacists, on the other hand, learn to know the mission of substances. They discover their healing relationship with human beings and familiarise themselves with a spiritual scientific understanding of health and illness. Furthermore, the joy in producing medicines, in the practical activity is reawoken in them.

And thus Rudolf Steiner's guiding verse, which he spoke at the end of a public lecture (GA 297) in the Stuttgart Waldorf School on 24 September 1919 for first time, is also suitable for our professional group:

Seek truly practical material life,
But seek it such that it does not insensitise you to the spirit at work in it.
Seek the spirit,
But seek it not in supersensory ecstasy, out of supersensory egoism,
But seek it
As you would use it selflessly in practical life, in the material world.

Apply the ancient principle:
"Spirit is never without matter, matter never without spirit" such that you say:
We want to do everything in the light of the spirit,
And we want to seek the light of the spirit such
That it develops warmth for us in our practical work.

Spirit guided by us into matter,
Matter on which we work to its revelation
Through which it shows the spirit within it;
Matter which receives revelation of the spirit through us,
Spirit which is driven towards matter through us,
They form the living existence
Which can bring humanity to achieve real progress,
To such progress which can only be longed for by the best in the profoundest depths of souls in our present time.

Rudolf Steiner[85]

The whole tone is one which challenges us, urging us to act with emphasis on the will. "Seek ..." "Apply ..." "We want ..." Such a search and implementation is based on an "ancient principle": "Spirit is ..." The words sound a warning not to seek the spirit in "supersensory ecstasy". The luciferic rejection of earthly working life is to be avoided, instead we should strive for the spiritual side of life with the goal to give warmth to everyday life, to our working life with spirit-borne thoughts. We use them to influence and penetrate earthly material existence so that it can show itself in its true spiritual aspect.

In order to turn a substance into a medicine, the pharmacist must accompany every manufacturing process, e.g. the potentisation process, with thoughts which carry healing within them. Substance is gradually freed from its material aspect and reveals the spirit which is at work in it. If we can succeed in this in the best possible way, progress is created for the health of the human being. This guiding verse calls on us to undertake our work with warmth and love carried by the spirit and can keep inspiring us to bring about such progress.

Research Council

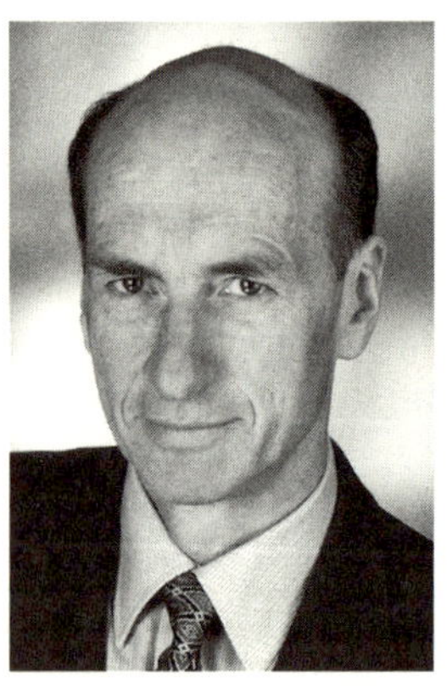

Dr med. Helmut Kiene
International Coordination of Research
helmut.kiene@ifaemm.de
www.dialogforum-pluralismusinder
medizin.de

After research on AM was given a clearly more professional form in the first seven years after the turn of the century, in parallel to the development of evidence-based medicine in conventional medicine, there was an additional significant perspective by the conclusion of the second septennium in the attempt at greater academisation. This path of academisation is now increasingly bearing fruit.

There are today more than 20 physicians who have obtained their habilitation in the context of AM, partly due to grants or funding for research projects. Meanwhile there are also various professorships which have AM reflected in their name: leading the way, the Gerhard Kienle Chair at Witten/Herdecke University is today called the "Chair of Medical Theory, Integrative and Anthroposophic Medicine"; the holder is Prof. Dr med. Peter Heusser. There are various professorships attached to this chair, including in this year a "Professorship for Integrative Neuromedicine with the focus on Anthroposophic Medicine" (Prof. Dr med. Wolfram Scharbrodt).

In the Netherlands the University of Applied Sciences Leiden has a professorship in "Anthroposophic Healthcare", the holder is Prof. Dr med. Erik Baars. An extraordinary professorship of anthroposophically extended medicine was established at the University of Bern in 2014 which was taken on by Prof. Dr med. Ursula Wolf. Additional similar steps towards academisation can be expected in the future.

The research activities outside universities are of course as important as ever alongside this extended university basis, particularly as they sometimes offer greater freedom with regard to positioning.

A leading research field in anthroposophic medicine continues to be research into mistletoe therapy with more than 1000 publications in scientific journals and over 150 clinical studies on the question of efficacy. It is however the case that until now most of these studies did not meet the formal quality standards demanded today.

We can obtain an idea of the breadth, diversity and dynamicism of research today when we realise that in the German-speaking countries there are meanwhile over 20 research facilities on anthroposophic medicine: they are at the medicine manufacturers Weleda, WALA, Helixor, Hiscia, Abnoba and Birken; the hospitals Herdecke, Research Institute Havelhöhe/FFIH, Filder Clinic Institute of Academic Research in Complementary and Integrative Medicine/ARCIM, Arlesheim, Richterswil as well as at the universities and higher education institutions Witten/Herdecke (chair), integrated supplementary studies in anthroposophic medicine; University Centre of Naturopathy and Research Centre at the University of Freiburg; IFAEMM Freiburg; Carus Institute Öschelbronn; Alanus University; IKOM Bern.

It will be important in future to set up increased numbers of research projects on the subjects of cognitive methodology, anthropology and training of anthroposophical cognitive skills.

International Coordination of Anthroposophic Medicine – School of Spiritual Science

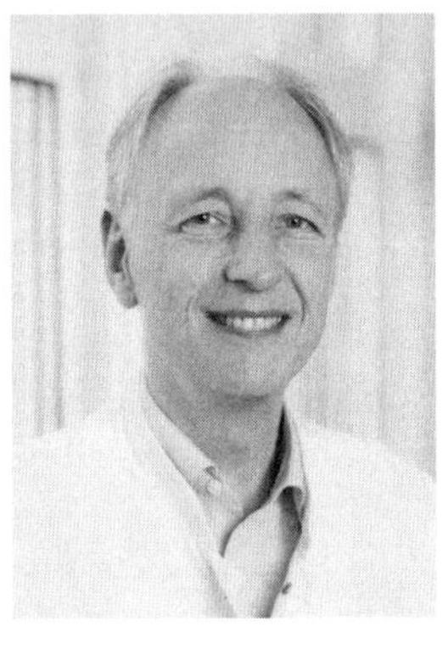

Dr med. Matthias Girke
International Coordination of Study in the School of Spiritual Science
Coordination of Anthromedics Project
matthias.girke@havelhoehe.de
www.havelhoehe.de

The path of knowledge of the School of Spiritual Science takes its specific form in the individual sections. This path, which aims to lead to true humanity and combine the spirit in the human being with the spirit in the world, is connected with the central questions of medicine and the art of healing.

Thus diagnosis in itself already requires the spiritual scientific dimension of the constitutional elements of the human being in order to be able to approach the being of the patient and determine the need for healing as well as the specific treatment. The latter must be examined not just with regard to its efficacy but beyond that poses the question as to what is "good" for the patient.

In each encounter with the patient the scientific question as to the appropriate treatment turns into the moral one "how do

I find the good?". Here guidelines will not help us any further; on the contrary, it requires the ability to reach an ethical decision through a meditative path of knowledge. After all, in the therapeutic relationship with the patient the threshold to the spiritual being of the other person with its challenges becomes real and demands that we deal with the numerous doubts and questions about meaning as we support the patient: rejection and "hate" of the disease "against which action has to be taken" and the various qualities of fear and anxiety which can occur both in the patient and the therapist.

The meditative path of knowledge is not separate from practice and life but fertilises our therapeutic work and everyday skills through the development of the capacity of therapeutic inspiration, deepening the relationship with the patient and his or her destiny as well as strengthening the therapeutically effective forces. The community-building environment of the Michael School is formed through the individual path of knowledge and the effort of will of the individual which takes effect down into the practical work.

The work of the School of Spiritual Science in the field of medicine deals with medical issues in conferences for those working therapeutically in the various professional groups. Another task is to support the development of the content of Anthroposophic Medicine and its presentation as well as representation in public.

This includes support for spiritual scientific research into the conceptions of diseases and therapeutic procedures as they are undertaken in the various work contexts of the therapeutic professions. The efficacy of their conceptions and results have to be examined through basic research and the various instruments of evaluative research.

The results of this work flow into the Anthromedics project. As the portal of Anthroposophic Medicine, its aim is to serve both the familiarisation with and entry into Anthroposophic Medicine and the deepening of its understanding of illness and treatment concepts. Currently it is essentially based on articles from *Merkurstab – Journal of Anthroposophic Medicine*, published by the Medical Section and Society of Anthroposophic Physicians in Germany (GAÄD). The latter will be available in full scope (articles since 1946) on publication in 2016.

A complete overview of Anthroposophic Medicine and its practical fields of life as well as the presentation of the individual specialist areas will also be published in future. The ongoing translation project aims to ensure that as many texts as possible are available not only in German, but also in English and Spanish.

The International Young Medics Forum

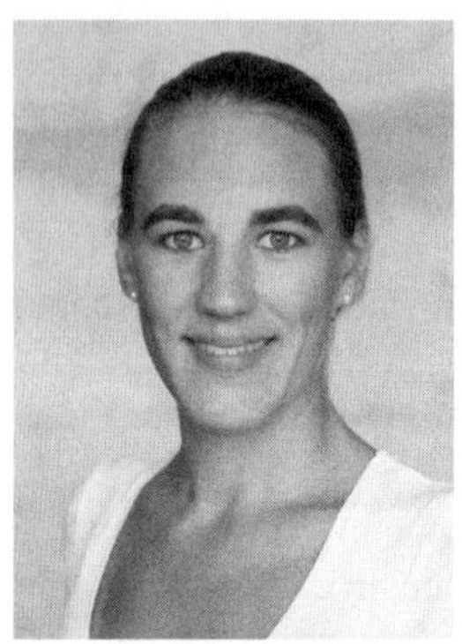

Anna Sophia Werthmann, physician
International Coordination of Young Medics Forum
anna.sophia.werthmann@jungmedizinerforum.org
www.jungmedizinerforum.org

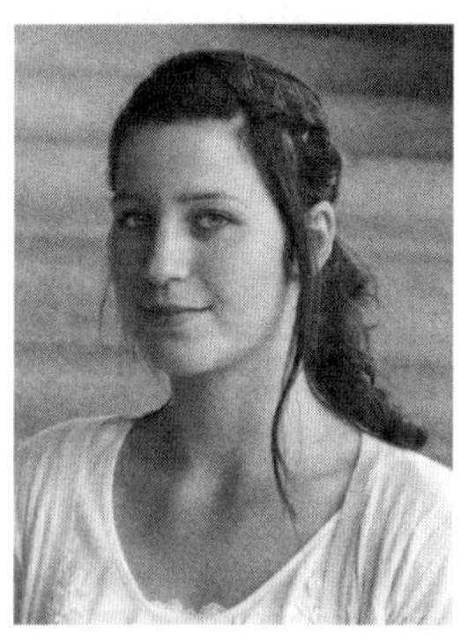

Tanja Geib, medical student
International Coordination of Young Medics Forum
tanja.geib@jungmedizinerforum.org
www.jungmedizinerforum.org

For the Young Medics Forum: Tanja Geib, Ann-Kristin Olk, Franziska Schüler, Anna Sophia Werthmann, Philipp Busche, Christoph Holtermann, Johannes Weinzirl, Paul Werthmann.

The origin of the Young Medics Forum: As a result of the concern to create an awareness of and build networks catering for the needs, initiatives and working groups of anthroposophic medical students, the "International Coordination of Student Work" formed in the Medical Section at the Goetheanum in 2003. In 2011 this developed into today's "Young Medics Forum" whose name was chosen on the one hand with a view to the socially creative work of Helene of Grunelius and on the other following on from the Young Physicians Course given by Rudolf Steiner – and thus also the meetings of young physicians held for many years at the Goetheanum.

The Young Medics Forum is organised in an independent, international and interdisciplinary way and is thus connected with the Medical Section of the School of Spiritual Science at the Goetheanum. Accordingly it is represented in the International Coordination of Anthroposophic Medicine (IKAM).

We are young medical students and physicians with an interest to Anthroposophic Medicine and as a forum wish to provide a meeting place which contributes to young people being able to realise their impulses. Our guiding principle in this context is the question: "How do I become a good physician?"

Collaboration: In the Young Medics Forum a small group of co-workers – surrounded by many people with initiative throughout the world – is engaged in a wide range of projects. The role of the co-workers can be characterised by continuous, committed collaboration. Their aim is to keep an overview of existing activities as well as an awareness of current needs and tasks. New co-workers are admitted in agreement with all co-workers. Decisions are taken jointly. Short-term decisions in the name of the Young Medics Forum can be taken by each co-worker individually on the basis of our guiding principles.

Each co-worker can work in any number of projects of the Young Medics Forum. The projects are each taken care of by one or several co-workers as well as other people with initiative outside this group. Tasks are distributed in accordance with the principle of initiative. Each person takes on the tasks they want to take on. Each new tasks that arrives is communicated. Tasks which have not yet been taken up are examined for their necessity. If it is identified as being necessary, it becomes a project of the Young Medics Forum. Tasks taken up out of independent initiative are much simpler to carry through than external obligations.

The principle of initiative has so far proved itself to be a good way of transforming obligations arising from a matter itself into an inner obligation. Not only have we learnt to develop initiative but we also had to learn to hand tasks over. It is part of life and all the questions it asks of us that we are occasionally taken to the limits of what we are capable of doing. For such cases there is agreement that this should be openly communicated. It happens repeatedly that we support or represent one another or help to carry the tasks of someone else for a time. Even the overall coordination is borne by various different people for certain periods. Initiative requires solidarity.

Meetings take place about twice a year to make awareness of one another and reaching agreement easier. Communication between meetings takes place by email, monthly telephone conferences and Internet-based project management software.

Public relations: A significant part of the Young Medics Forum is to network anthroposophically interested young people and provide information about conferences and seminars. This frequently happens in cooperation with other initiatives such as for example the GAÄD (Society of Anthroposophic Physicians in Germany) Academy.

The Young Medics Forum sends out a circular email about four times a year which provides information about current activities and events. In order to support young people and make access to Anthroposophic Medicine easier for them, the Young Medics Forum in cooperation with the GAÄD and the Initiative für Ausbildung in Anthroposophischer Medizin e.V. (Initiative for Training in Anthroposophic Medicine) has developed a package for students and assistant physicians which includes, among other things, a reduced GAÄD membership fee, a *Merkurstab* subscription and reduced conference fees.

The website of the Young Medics Forum (www.jungmedizinerforum.org) additionally serves as a contact and information point. A calendar is maintained there, among other things, which tries to reflect all anthroposophic medical events so that one can obtain an overview both of all activities and of events such as the introductory seminar, the study week, etc.

Internationality: The Whitsun conference "Enlightening the heart" in May 2013 was the first international conference organised by the Young Medics Forum. During the conference there were daily meetings on international collaboration so that we were able to form an initial picture of the questions, ideas and concerns in the other countries. The framework conditions (e.g. the existence of training centres, the possibility of prescribing anthroposophic medicines) are different everywhere.

It became clear that it was everyone's wish to be in contact with one another to reflect on questions of content and organisation. We would like to support people with initiative in projects in their home countries with the experience we have gathered through our activity. We want to help young people to come together in the different countries to take on the coordinating work in their region.

The 2013 Whitsun conference also revealed the value of personal encounters. In this context we are also planning further international meetings, e.g. within the framework of the annual conference of the Medical Section at the Goetheanum.

Interdisciplinarity: How can the various nursing, therapeutic and medical professions work together in a way that serves the well-being of patients? What does each professional group contribute to the healing process and in which way? These and similar questions have been reflected upon since the student coordination was founded and are still thought about just as intensively in the Young Medics Forum. Out of the concern to enable and develop good reciprocal perception, respect and new forms of collaboration among the young generation, there have for some years been interdisciplinary conferences of the "Forum Asklepios".

In 2013 these questions were a central subject at the Whitsun conference "Enlightening the heart". Since then new "young" connections have developed. Some of them are attached to the Young Medics Forum so that the existing infrastructures can be used, or they are organised independently. Starting from the

Young Medics Forum, we want to support these initiatives as much as we can and further cultivate the collaboration among the medical professional groups.

Financing of the coordination: In order to keep the organisational costs for the Young Medics Forum as low as possible, it was decided not to establish an independent legal entity. The collaboration with the Initiative für Ausbildung in Anthroposophischer Medizin e.V. offers the opportunity for such a social and legal base. In addition, the Initiative provides the financial resources required by the Young Medics Forum so it can organise its own meetings, projects and similar things. The financial resources of the Initiative come from foundations, sponsors and individual donors.

Fields of initiative

Young medics meetings: There is regular work on the content of themes in the "Young Physicians Course".[86] The young medics meetings are organised by the Young Medics Forum and represent an opportunity for young medical students and physicians to meet one another – with space to get to know one another, exchange thoughts and ideas and, above all, ask questions. The focus of the work and approach vary depending on the composition of the preparatory group concerned.

Students: How can I learn something about the nature of health and illness, the will to heal and the medicines themselves without being engaged in a therapeutic process with my patients on a daily basis? As students we are mostly not linked to an anthroposophic clinic, often alone in a city, without connection to an anthroposophical work context. In this context we see our task as supporting the training route of each individual person. This can range from personal meetings and discussions to creating networks among students and working groups, facilitating clinical traineeships and research work as well as spreading information about seminars and conferences. We help working groups to establish or deepen themselves and it is our aim to support each young person on their individual path.

Young physicians: The question as to our own training to become a good physician continues to be with us also after we have concluded our studies. Many young physicians seek such a position in an anthroposophical clinic to become acquainted with the practical application of the medicines and how to deal with patients on the basis of the anthroposophical image of the human being. We wish to support this desire and strengthen social cohesion through exchange opportunities.

Some clinics already have good and structured further training provision in the field of mainstream medicine as well as Anthroposophic Medicine. In collaboration with other organisations and establishments of Anthroposophic Medicine, we want to help to improve the working conditions of young physicians who have an interest in Anthroposophic Medicine.

Facilitating research work: There are numerous opportunities in the context of Anthroposophic Medicine for writing a diploma or doctoral dissertation. The range of content and methodology is very wide in this context. Examples might be literature reviews in the field of the theory/philosophy of medicine (for example on body-soul interaction), experimental work (basic research into phytotherapy, cell biology, homoeopathy), artistic therapeutic studies, medicine studies (e.g. on mistletoe therapy), qualitative research (questionnaires, interviews, discourse analyses), single case descriptions (e.g. in the sense of Cognition Based Medicine), work on medical anthropology or organology (e.g. in the sense of a Goethean phenomenology) up to and including more profound anthroposophical questions and research methods. Behind all these fields there are different people, institutes and universities which we are happy to facilitate.

Newsletter: The newsletter appears about once a year in printed form and essentially consists of readers' contributions. With the newsletter we wish to provide space for an exchange of views and dialogue about current questions and subjects as well as reporting to each other about personal experiences at conferences, seminars, working groups and clinics.

Inner development in our own profession – the path with the mantras of the Young Physicians Course

Philipp Busche, René Ebersbach

A total of five "young medics meetings" took place from 2011 to 2013. An integral part of the meetings is formed by joint work on the content and mantras of the so-called Young Physicians Course.[87] Despite the intensive study of these meditations, it is difficult to put anything down on paper which has meaning, and above all validity, beyond the moment of the meetings. Access to the mantras, their use and thoughts about them are as diverse as the young people who come together for the meetings. Many of the thoughts included here arose in joint conversation at the young medics meetings. We would like to use this opportunity to thank our friends warmly for their input.

The ambit of the mantras

The book title *Understanding Healing. Meditative Reflections on Deepening Medicine through Spiritual Science* at the same time characterises its content.

It is noteworthy that seven word and verse meditations, so-called mantras, occupy the central position in the lectures. The lectures are full of information to help the understanding of the content and context of these mantras. Rudolf Steiner precedes some mantras with other exercises. They explain how to use the respective meditation or enable a similar experience by other means, thus for example the three-part plant observation in accordance with Sal, Mercury and Sulphur in the fourth lecture of the Christmas course,[88] or the exercise with the gold leaf in the eighth lecture.[89] The introductions give the person using these exercises much help to study their content. They can use the supplementary exercises to deepen the practice of the mantras.

The effect of the mantras

Every meditation develops an ability in the soul. One of the prerequisites of anthroposophical meditation is to work to understand the effect of the meditation concerned in order to remain inwardly free. Starting from such a basic understanding of anthroposophical training, it was an essential work stage for us to seek out these effects in the numerous statements in the lectures.

Anyone who studies the lectures in the Young Physicians Course will be aware of the wealth of suggestions they contain for our meditative life. Thus the following reflections will only be able to look at a single aspect from the perspective chosen by us of the effect, something which by itself does not, of course, do justice to the complexity of these descriptions. But even the findings obtained in this way appear to us to be of such value that they can encourage us in our own inner work. We are aware that the effects of the mantras are many-faceted and various. We make no claim to completeness here. On the contrary, the close connection between these meditations and questions arising from our studies and everyday medical life was a particular discovery for us.

An overview

"The warmth meditation ...":

Preparation: How do I find the good?

1. Can I think the good?

   I cannot think the good.
   Thinking is brought about by my etheric body.
   My etheric body works in the fluid of my body.
   Therefore I do not find the good in the fluid of the body.

2. Can I feel the good?

   I can indeed feel the good; however, it is not made present by me if I only feel it.

Feeling is brought about by my astral body.
My astral body works in the aeriform of my body.
Therefore in the aeriform of my body I cannot find the good that exists through me.

3. Can I will the good?

I can will the good.
Willing is brought about by my I.
My I works in the warmth ether of my body.
Therefore in the warmth I can physically realise the good.

I feel my humanity in my warmth

1. I feel light in my warmth.
(Take care that this sensation of light emerges in the region where the physical heart lies)

2. I feel, sounding, world substance in my warmth.
(Take care that the specific sensation of tone goes from the lower body towards the head but spreading out into the whole body)

3. I feel in my head cosmic life stirring in my warmth.
(Take care that the specific sensation of life spreads from the head to the whole body)

Rudolf Steiner[90]

"Helene (von Grunelius) complained that it was impossible for her to follow the advice about the 'notebook' because it was impossible to know whether what one wrote on the right (spiritual scientific) side was correct. Rudolf Steiner responded: 'Doesn't matter, you yourself will make corrections over time. Furthermore, you can send me your notebooks. But if you want to obtain greater assurance, I can give you a meditation.' And he gave her the warmth meditation ..."[91] This meditation was given before the Young Physicians Course and in a certain sense forms its prelude. It was a help for the "double-entry bookkeeping" and a path to seeing the etheric Christ.[92]

Double-entry bookkeeping is particularly important at the start of our studies since it is intended to help establish the right relationship between natural science and spiritual science. The second statement creates an arc to a high ideal of physicianhood. Thus the warmth meditation encompasses the whole developmental path of the physician, starting during our studies and great vista at the same time.

"Ye healing spirits ...":

Ye healing spirits
You unite
With sulphur's blessing
In the ethereal fragrance;

You come to life
In Mercury's upward striving,
Dewdrop
Of growing
And becoming.

You come to rest
In the earth salt
Which nourishes the root
In the soil. –

I will unite
The knowledge of my soul
With fire of the flower's fragrance;

I will bestir
The life of my soul
On the glistening drop of leafy morning;

I will make strong the being of my soul
With the hardening salt

With which the earth
With loving care nurtures the root. –

Rudolf Steiner[93]

In studying medicine today, the knowledge which is taught can be experienced as lifeless and abstract. Such knowledge does not lead to an interest in the specific patient; it has been shown that the capacity for empathy of students clearly falls in the course of their studies.[94] Here the meditative study of these mantras and going into nature is of help. "That is to say, you will start [...] to bring life into your medical knowledge, to look at nature and people in such a way that healing comes to you out of the strong impulse [...] to help."[95] Living knowledge and the capacity for empathy, that is to say the intention to render assistance, belong together.

"See in thy Soul power of radiance ...":

See in thy soul
    Power of radiance
Feel in thy body
    Might of heaviness
In the power of radiance
    Shines spirit-I
In the might of heaviness
    God's spirit works with strength
Yet shall not
    Power of radiance
Grasp
    Might of heaviness
Nor
    Might of heaviness
Penetrate
    Power of radiance
For if power of radiance grasps
    Might of heaviness
And if might of heaviness penetrates
    Power of radiance

Soul and body
    Will be bound to their ruin
In cosmic confusion.

Rudolf Steiner[96]

"You see, through such reflections you will get to those characteristics of a substance which are required for therapy".[97] Beyond knowledge of the illness, and as actually to be expected by the content, the meditative study of this mantra can lead to the development of the ability to identify medicines and an eye for "the therapeutic element of eurythmy therapy".[98] It was astounding for us that we meditate on the illness and thereby obtain the ability to identify medicines.

"It was in ancient times …":

It was in ancient times,
That there lived in the souls of initiates
Powerfully the thought that
By nature every human being is sick.
And education was seen
As a healing process
Which, as they matured,
Gave children the health
To be complete human beings in life.

Rudolf Steiner[99]

This mantra is the fourth one in the chronological sequence and takes a special position by virtue of the fact alone that it was not given within the course but was sent out in the newsletter between the Christmas and Easter course. The information about its action is restricted to a single sentence. "It is a good thing to allow such powerful thoughts […] to stand before our soul if we want to prepare the soul in the right inner mood to grasp the healing effects."[100] If we have a therapeutic idea and prescribe a medicine in the assumption that it is the right thing for the patient, then this meditation helps to perceive its effects.

This ability, which can only gradually be developed as an aspiring physician, serves to evaluate the therapy.

"Behold, what is joined in the cosmos ...":

Behold, what is joined in the cosmos,
Thou feelest the forming of the human being.
– this in connection with the moon.
Behold, all that moves thee in air,
– for example in the respiration or blood circulation –
Thou wilt experience the human being's ensoulment.
– this is in connection with the sun.
Behold, what is changed in the earthly,
– primarily those things which also bring death to human beings –
Thou wilt discern the spiritualising of the human being.
– this in connection with Saturn.

Behold, what is joined in the cosmos,
Thou feelest the forming of the human being.

Behold, all that moves thee in air,
Thou wilt experience the human being's ensoulment.

Behold, what is changed in the earthly,
Thou wilt discern the spiritualising of the human being.

Rudolf Steiner[101]

The clear structure and the content of this mantra make its effect obvious: "[...] then you will learn to look into the human being."[102] "In this way you will discover what is built into the human being from the cosmos, from the surroundings of the earth, of earthly forces." "[...] if we thoroughly want to understand the human being, specifically, if we want to understand them with regard to curing them [...]",[103] then we develop the ability in the meditative study of this mantra for a diagnosis which takes the action of cosmic and earthly forces in the patient into account.

"Feel in fever's measure ...":

Feel in fever's *measure*
Saturn's gift of spirit
Feel in the pulse's *count*
The *sun's* soul strength
Feel in the *weight* of matter
The forming power of the *moon:*
Then you will see in your will to heal
Also the need to be healed of the *earthly* human being.

Rudolf Steiner[104]

The outer taking of a person's temperature, counting their pulse and weighing matter should change in that we turn our inner attention to the cosmic relationship of human beings. Through the meditative study of the mantra "[...] you will obtain an intuition of what you should do".[105] Beyond understanding of the human being and diagnosis, we will recognise what can be done therapeutically. Beyond the general knowledge of what characterises a medicine, we can identify what will help in this individual case. Another effect is described as: "[...] the person penetrating these things with their heart, their soul has the best opportunity to perceive in the ill person what has come across from previous incarnations, or at least to have a sense of it."[106] Thus this mantra provides the skill for actual practical work in looking after patients today.

"Push forward infancy ...":

Push forward infancy
Into childhood
And childhood
Into youth.
To you will appear condensed
Human etheric existence
Behind physical being –

Push back the density of old age

Into the period of human maturity
And maturity
Into youthful life.
To you will resound in cosmic tones
Human soul activity
Out of etheric life.

Rudolf Steiner[107]

Two skills are to be practised in this general observation of the human being which connect the specific professional schooling path of the physician directly with the general schooling of anthroposophy. If we meditate on this mantra, "[...] then there really is born in you" – in working with the first section – "the imagination of the human etheric body; the imagination of the human etheric body is born relatively fast".[108] In working with the second part "[we] obtain an impression of the astral part of the human being".[109] The last of the seven mantras thus leads to an understanding of the supersensory part of the human being in a general way. This closes the arc to the warmth meditation in a surprising way; after all, a vision of the etheric Christ presupposes a knowledge of the etheric.

The path with the mantras of the Young Physicians Course

Looked at from the perspective of their action, the individual mantras thus coalesce into a meaningful composition. Surprisingly, the effects which have been described and which we worked on together did not always correspond with our expectations. In chronological order, the mantras can help to develop the following skills:

- making our studies more comprehensive through double-entry bookkeeping;
- enlivening knowledge and developing the will to heal;
- enabling understanding of medicines;
- therapy evaluation;
- being able to find the right diagnosis;
- finding the right therapy in the individual case and starting to

be able to draw up a diagnosis of the human constitutional elements.

These skills are the core competences of the medical profession. In working inwardly with these mantras, our own schooling obtains great relevance for our practical work.

Our joint work in the young medics meetings has encouraged us to continue working with the mantras. And so we hope that the beauty of their composition and their practical relevance will also encourage other people to work with them.

Clinic Coordination and the development of the Anthromed label

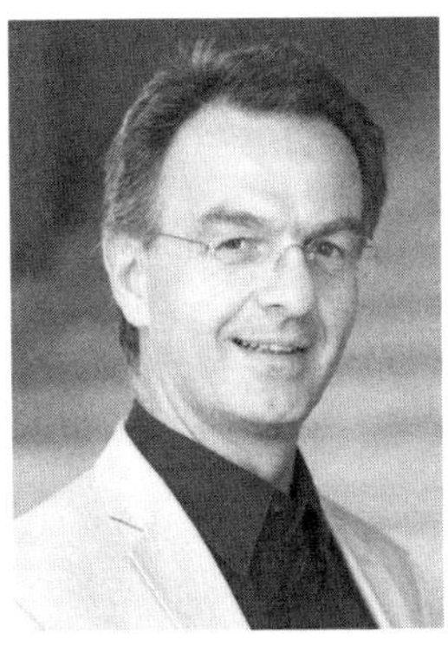

Dr math. Andreas Jäschke
International Coordination of Anthroposophic Clinics
andreas.jaeschke@klinik-arlesheim.ch
www.klinik-arlesheim.ch

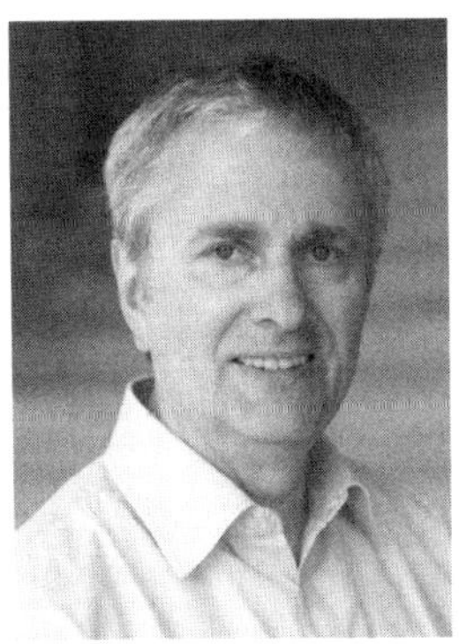

Dr med. Roland Bersdorf
Coordinator of the AnthroMed® label within the IKAM collegium
roland.bersdorf@anthromed.net
www.anthromed.net

The twenty-five members of the Association of Anthroposophic Clinics come together twice each year to meet one another and exchange views in a plenary meeting. In 2005, nine clinics belonging to the association founded the company "gemeinnützige AnthroMed GmbH" as an instrument for performing various operational tasks. The subject of creating a label within Anthroposophic Medicine has been worked on in close cooperation with the Medical Section since as long ago as 2004. Branding and the development of a label are essentially about condensing spiritual aspects – issues of identity, mission, etc. – into an instrument and thus making them usable in an entrepreneurial context.

It was agreed with IKAM that the clinics would actively advance this process and that it should be structured in such an open way that other professional groups, where interested, could participate in this brand-forming process. In 2007 the "AnthroMed®" label was registered. There is a list of criteria and procedures for obtaining the brand rights.

The clinics as shareholders of AnthroMed GmbH are meanwhile all certified. The process of recertification has started since then. To this extent this instrument has proved its suitability for daily use.

Meanwhile the quality mark "AnthroMed®" has been developed further for use beyond the clinical field. Thus there are currently brand agreements for the professional fields of eurythmy therapy and pharmacy. Others are in preparation, particularly in the international field – where national adjustments have to be made.

A further central range of tasks is the support of member establishments of the Association and clinical initiatives. That includes enquiries from existing hospitals who in the course of general structural reforms are interested in some provision falling within the framework of Anthroposophic Medicine. The factors limiting this task are the completely inadequate financial possibilities for strategic involvement. Marginalisation of clinical Anthroposophic Medicine because of insufficient growth capacity remains a very grave threat.

Another and exceptionally important project concerns the training of anthroposophic physicians, something that is being worked on together with the medical associations.

The social form and structure of collaboration in an anthroposophic hospital is another central field of work of the clinics alongside the branding. We still have the concept of the "community hospital" from Gerhard Kienle which places the focus on "togetherness". But the aspect of "leadership" is becoming ever more crucial, not least because our hospitals have to move in an increasingly competitive environment and thus the entrepreneurial character is emerging every more clearly.

At the same time there is the spiritual and social challenge of preparing the social context of an establishment as a whole in the same way as a medicine, because a key special feature of our facilities lies in the action of the healing forces coming from this dimension, something which needs to be developed further.

Anthroposophic nursing

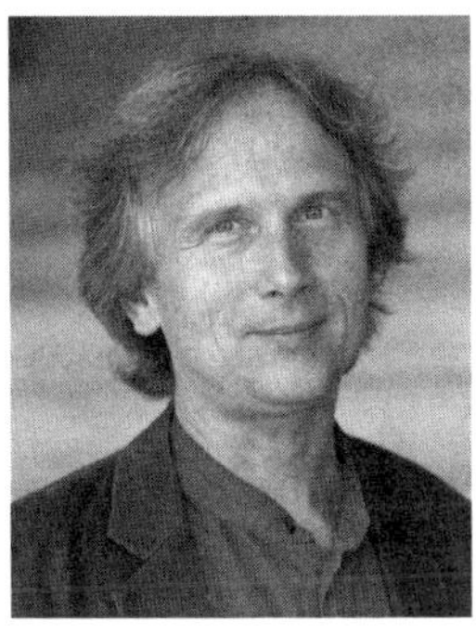

Rolf Heine, Nurse
Coordination of Anthroposophic Nursing
r.heine@filderklinik.de
www.vfap.de

What is the contribution of anthroposophic nursing in the system of Anthroposophic Medicine?

Nursing is part of all areas of the life from birth to death. Caring for children, ill people, people with disabilities or the elderly often requires professional support. Three sentences describe the nature and task of nursing: "nursing enables illness", "nursing lends permanence to therapy" and "without nursing all the gains of culture fall back into a state of meaningless nature".

How many anthroposophic nurses are active worldwide?

About 3000 professional nurses are working on the basis of anthroposophy in 16 countries on all continents, with the focus on German-speaking Europe. The overwhelming number is employed in anthroposophically oriented hospitals, facilities for the elderly, out-patient nursing services, medical practices or nursing practices. A significant number, which is however difficult to estimate, is working in conventional establishments in the health system.

How is the association of anthroposophic nurses organised? How is it financed?

There are nine national associations for anthroposophic nursing which have come together in the International Forum for Anthroposophic Nursing (IFAN). In addition, all professional nurses can become co-workers in IFAN who represent an initiative in the field of anthroposophic nursing. The forum consists of approx. 60 nurses from all over the world who meet once a year at the Goetheanum. A coordinator is chosen for three years by the Forum. A management group manages business together with the coordinator.

In 2014 the International Council of Anthroposophic Nursing Associations (ICANA) was founded as the association of the national professional associations of anthroposophic nursing. As a registered association, it is the legal organ of IFAN.

The Quality in Anthroposophic Nursing (QAN) agency runs approval proceedings for training provisions in anthroposophic nursing worldwide on behalf of IFAN.

This has created a threefold structure in anthroposophic nursing: IFAN is the forum for the exchange of views and initiative, an organ of the cultural life. ICANA represents the legal business of the movement internally and externally. QAN provides services for the co-workers and organisations of anthroposophic nursing.

The Forum and its leadership organs is financed through contributions from the national associations as well as currently through a sponsored secondment of the coordinator.

How are the modes of work and responsibility structures described in this book practiced in anthroposophic nursing?

Membership is founded exclusively in the purpose to represent an anthroposophic nursing initiative. Admission to the Forum takes place following consultation with the coordinator. The forms of working together are set out in rules of procedure which are the result of a joint development process and which consider themselves to be connected with the responsibility structures of the Medical Section.

The Forum, the management group and the coordinator have taken on responsibility for the worldwide development of anthroposophic nursing as part of the medical system of anthroposophy. This includes taking care of specialist and professional development through training, further training and advanced training; the agreement of standards for the reciprocal recognition of training qualifications; consultancy in specialist and professional policy questions; the development of relations with other professional and task fields in the Medical Section; and also the cultivation of work on the esotericism of the profession and involvement in the First Class of the School of Spiritual Science.

What training, further training and advanced training provisions are there?

There are five state-recognised nursing schools worldwide. The problem of finding new nurses for the hospitals and care establishments has been recognised and joint efforts to attract recruits to these establishments have begun. There is further training in anthroposophic nursing in nine countries worldwide.

How is the spiritual substance cultivated?

At the core of the anthroposophic nursing movement are five meditative verses given by Rudolf Steiner, the so-called "nurses' verse", the "Find yourself in Light" meditation, the three meditations from the so-called "Samaritan course" and the so-called "therapeutic emblem". In addition, meditations which Rudolf

Steiner specifically gave to physicians – the so-called "warmth meditation" and the verse "Seek in fever's measure" – have a particular connection with the nurse's inner path.

Both these meditations are therefore especially suited to creating a common spiritual bond between physicians and nurses. Of the meditations mentioned here, only the nurses' verse was specifically intended for the professional group of nurses. The rest were given in other contexts but have a strong inner connection with nursing. Ita Wegman was given the nurses' verse by Rudolf Steiner on 2 December 1923 with the express instruction only to give it to the nurses when good collaboration existed and a new community had been formed.

As a result the verse was given to seven selected nurses who were members of the First Class of the School of Spiritual Science on occasion of the first nurses course in 1925. This group was at the same time admitted to the Medical Section as a "subdivision". Until it was published in the 1990s, the nurses' verse was circulated solely amongst members of the First Class of the School of Spiritual Science and was used meditatively for developing heart forces in an individual, the professional community and nursing practice.

After it was published, those who work with this meditation agreed to engage with it every Sunday morning in awareness of a worldwide spiritual bond between nurses, and to include in this meditation the dead who had lived and worked in the spirit of this meditation. All who work with the nurses' verse are invited to join this bond of spiritual practice.

Within the heart there lives
In radiant light
The human will to help.
Within the heart there works
In warmth-giving power
The human force of love.
Then let us bear
The soul's whole will
In heart-warmth
And heart-light
Then we work to heal

Those in need of healing
Through God's sense of grace.

Rudolf Steiner[110]

The meditation "Find yourself in Light" which Rudolf Steiner gave was for many years practiced at the beginning of the day by Ita Wegman with nurses at the Clinical and Therapeutic Institute. Work with this meditation enhances the capacity to awaken in the etheric and imaginative world, and to strengthen our I awareness in this continually transforming, dissolving and recondensing world.

Find yourself in Light
With your own soul's tone;
And tone disperses,
Becomes colour-form
    In the Light –
Light – Divinities – Being.

Tone disappeared
Restored again within him
    Speaking through him:
        You are
Your own tone in the light of the world
    Sound illuminating
    Illuminate sounding.

Rudolf Steiner[111]

Rudolf Steiner introduced the meditations in the Samaritan course a few days after the outbreak of the First World War as the focus of a series of four lectures. The aim of this course was to give a practical introduction to emergency first aid. The course was divided into a practical part with wound care and bandaging techniques, and another part with lectures on the esoteric background to wound healing, empathic help and the causes of violent conflicts. Since then, the two mantric verses "Well up o blood" and "As long as thou dost feel the pain" have been an important part of nurses' esoteric schooling in dealing with wounds and pain.

Well up o blood
And in the welling work;
Quickening muscles,
Quicken the seeds;
May loving care
Of a warming heart
Be healing breath.

Rudolf Steiner[112]

As long as *thou* dost feel the pain
That avoids me
Is Christ unrecognised,
Working in the World-Being;
For the spirit only remains weak
When solely in its own body
It has the power to feel pain.

Rudolf Steiner[113]

The third verse of the Samaritan course turns to the folk spirit and points to the relationship between individual suffering and the suffering of communities, e.g. in connection with wars or natural disasters.

Thou spirit of my earthly realm,
Reveal the light of your age
To the soul gifted with Christ,
That in striving it can find you
In the choir of the spheres of peace,
Sounding the praise and might
Of human meaning in Christ devotion.

Rudolf Steiner[114]

The so-called therapeutic emblem was based on a design which

Rudolf Steiner made during the First World War. Helene Röchling gave it to nurses at the military hospital she founded as acknowledgement of their work.

The emblem, with the inscription "Blessed be the helpers of healing" shows the rays of the sun shining down on a pair of receiving hands towards which a single hand is inclining. A snake rises up between the radiating sun and the receiving hands as a symbol of knowledge and healing. The emblem is a pictorial meditation expressing the effect of "industrious love". The emblem became the model for the logo of several national anthroposophic nursing associations.

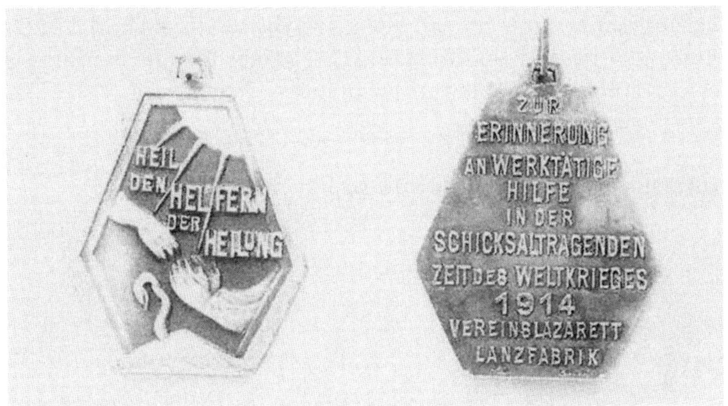

Therapeutic emblem
Logo of the Association for Anthroposophic Nursing

The meditation "Feel in fever's measure" was given to physicians attending the so-called Young Physicians Course.[115] Measuring a patient's temperature and weight, and taking their pulse – daily nursing tasks – are connected in this meditation with the whole of world evolution.

Practicing this meditation initially draws our attention to the sensory perception of the body and from there, mediated by the categories of measure, number and weight, penetrates through to the world's evolutionary laws. The meditation necessitates familiarising oneself with the fundamentals of world evolution. It is, on the one hand, a stimulus for studying spiritual science and, on the other, it leads lofty thoughts into the depths of sensory perception. The meditating person thus works on a key motif of nursing and connects this with the physician's will to heal.

The so-called warmth meditation marking the beginning of the physician's esoteric schooling was passed by the physician Karl König also to non-medical colleagues in the Camphill Community. There in particular it lives also among nurses as a special heart centre of their meditative work. The meditation is thematically connected with the nurses' verse. The nurses' verse works pictorially with the motif of warmth and focuses on the heart organ. The warmth meditation awakens forces of thinking and transforms them into an organ of perception for the streams of warmth ether in the human being and the world. Its initial question – "How do I find the good?" – makes this meditation the ethical foundation of anthroposophic medicine.

International Coordination of Psychotherapy

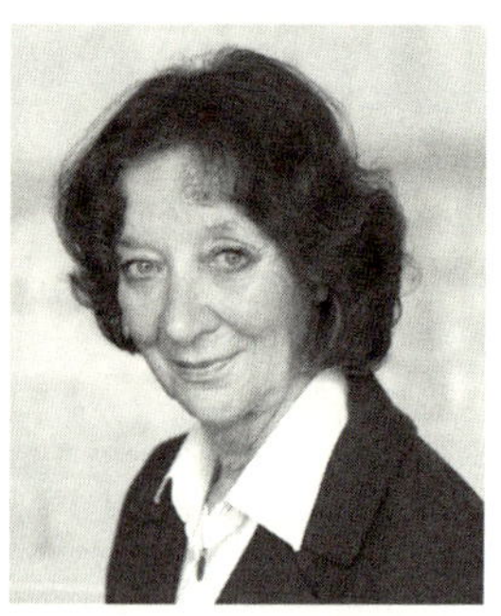

Henriette Dekkers, psychologist / psychotherapist
International Coordination of Psychotherapy
dekkers.appel@planet.nl
www.medsektion-goetheanum.org

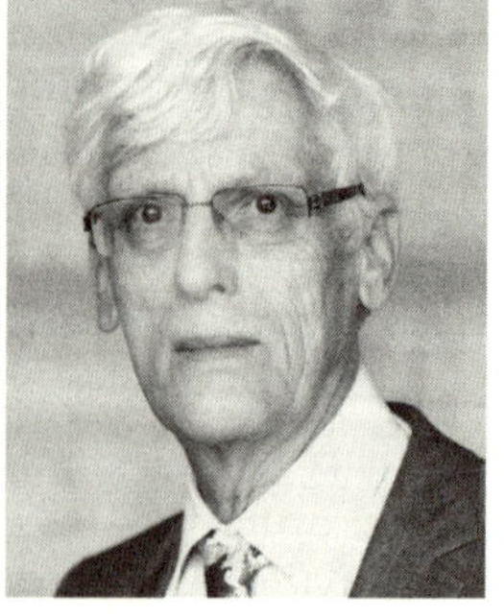

Ad Dekkers, psychologist/psychotherapist
International Coordination of Psychotherapy
dekkers.appel@planet.nl
www.medsektion-goetheanum.org

The original impulse of anthroposophically oriented psychotherapy

This is dated to about 1975 and from the beginning bore the hallmark of research. Rudolf Steiner – because he was never asked – developed neither special courses nor special training for psychotherapists. As a consequence the work and research activities of the first initiative group in Germany and the Netherlands created the basics for an extension of the diagnostic and treatment methods applied by psychiatrists, psychotherapists and physicians working in psychotherapy and general practice. Such basic research into and the investigation of the presentation of psychopathology, something that keeps changing over time, continue to be the focus of the work of this professional group.

1973: Prof. Dr med. Bernard Lievegoed initiated a working group for psychiatry and psychotherapy in the Netherlands and in 1978 undertook the first three-year post-doc advanced training, culminating in his book "Der Mensch an der Schwelle" (Man on the Threshold).

1979: Dr med. Paul von der Heide (Filder Clinic, Germany) founded the Institute for Anthroposophically Oriented Psychotherapy together with, among others, Dr med. Werner Priever, Dr med. Käthe Weizsäcker and Dr med. Hertha Lauer. Other key colleagues joined, including Dr med. Dieter Beck and Dr med. Hugo Solms (Switzerland).

Over the decades, the work of both initiative groups focused on the following foundations:

Spiritual schooling path for psychological and medical psychotherapists and psychiatrists, specifically with regard to subjects relating to the threshold to the spiritual world and the guardians of the threshold. Since 1991 this work has additionally taken place in the international conferences of the School of Spiritual Science in Dornach.

- Research on forms and ways of anthroposophic psychotherapeutic diagnosis, therapy and talk systematics.
- Pastoral-medical, constitutional, organ-psychiatric and karmic perspectives on psychiatric diagnosis and problems.

- Psychiatric-medical medication.
- Conventional medical psychotherapeutic diagnosis extended through practical and anthroposophical knowledge of the human being; treatment and prognostics based on joint research and clinical case reports.

The basic research into and investigation of the presentation of psychopathology, something that keeps changing over time, also serves other objectives:

1. Engaging in soul and spiritual training and conventional medical training with regard to changing psychopathology and

2. together updating guidelines for post-doc advanced training to the spiritual and conventional current state of medicine.

As an example we can cite the qualitative and quantitative increase in psychopathologies since the Second World War. Then there is the increase in identity problems (personality disorders – specifically borderline disorders), both a quantitative and qualitative increase in threshold phenomena, a quantitative increase in the problem of hetero- and auto-aggression, a growing quantum of anxiety-aggression-depression comorbidity and the inescapable problem of drug addiction. The change in the human constitution should also be mentioned, together with the growing problem area of the small child (incl. attention deficits, hyperactivity, learning disorders, autism spectrum problems, pervasive developmental disorders not otherwise specified).

The wish for anthroposophically oriented or based psychotherapy is growing constantly, as is the demand for training and assistance in corresponding initiatives.

Difference between psychiatry, psychosomatics and psychotherapy

The pathogenesis of psychiatric clinical pictures is closely connected with organ-related clinical pictures in patients. The psychosomatic clinical pictures tend to be based on chronic traumatisation in early childhood or are related to life-threatening shocking events. We refer to psychogenic physical pain and stress. Whereas psychiatric treatment is fundamentally based on

– in sequence – medication, treatment procedures based on the human constitutional elements, exercises and anthroposophic psychodidactics, the focus in psychotherapeutic practice is on processual development based on the diagnosis of the human constitutional elements and psychotherapeutic treatment of the threefold and fourfold human being with their biographical disorders and traumatisation.

Biography work

The work of the biographical therapeutic counsellor is oriented towards conversation, self-knowledge, biographical knowledge and self-control, counselling and help in crises and life events. In Britain, counsellors also engaged in psychiatric support.

The focus of biography work is on creative "steermanship" in the biographical ductus; here intact ego functions are essentially assumed with the help of which the ego human being can in principle manage the tasks of metamorphosis of the seven-year rhythms and their reflections in the biography.

Organisational structures

On 15 September 2012, the association "International Federation of Anthroposophic Psychotherapy Associations" (IFAPA) was founded in Dornach under Swiss law. It was established in the course of the International Medical Conference at the Goetheanum. The conference theme was "Psychiatry, psychosomatics and psychotherapy".

The Federation's members are countries in which there is already a society for anthroposophic psychotherapy: the Netherlands, Italy, Brazil, Germany, India, England, Spain, Argentina, the USA and Israel. Co-founders present who at the time of establishment did not yet have an official national society were Switzerland, Chile, Russia, Columbia and Mexico. There was great pleasure in having established connections throughout the world.

Core elements of the esoteric and exoteric organisation of IFAPA

The following core elements of the Federation – set out in the preamble – regarding its goals, co-responsibility towards the physical and spiritual world, membership and code of professional ethics are important.

- Anthroposophic psychotherapy is based both on modern academic and professional knowledge as well as the spiritual science developed by Rudolf Steiner which sees human beings in their interrelationships as a physical, psychological, spiritual and social individual.
- As such, anthroposophic psychotherapy is professionally based in the "School of Spiritual Science of the Medical Section".
- The methods of anamnesis, diagnosis, treatment and healing reflect this dimension in a differentiated way.
- These goals take account of the findings of spiritual science and academic research for which both spiritual and academic foundations are used in the professional training and continuous professional development of psychotherapists.
- In addition, the following is taken into account:
  - the physical, physiological, psychological and spiritual development of the child – in belonging to both worlds, earthly and spiritual – is considered in the context of their social ties;
  - the development of the human being as an individual during their lifetime;
  - the development of humanity as a whole;
  - the historical connection with world events in the light of the spirit of our time.

Membership of the Federation

Ordinary members of the International Federation (IFAPA) are national societies and associations whose goal consists of supporting and practising anthroposophically extended psychotherapy. Ordinary members are represented by two delegates.

The public purpose of the Federation is

- the representation of the national societies for anthroposophic psychotherapy and the coordination of their activities which are of international importance;
- assistance in promoting continuing professional development and securing a legal basis for professional standards, inter-country recognition as well as the development of research goals;
- assistance and support in the promotion of professional ethical principles as well as respect for our fellow human beings and the freedom of the individual.

Purpose – objectives – professional ethics

The International Federation of Anthroposophic Psychotherapy Associations (IFAPA) pursues the following goals:

- Representation of the national societies for anthroposophic psychotherapy within the meaning of the preamble at an international level.
- Coordination of the activities of international importance for the national societies.
- Providing mutual assistance for the members of IFAPA to promote national post-graduate basic training and advanced training as continuing professional development; here quality and qualification are assured through nationally recognised and internationally valid certification, and at national level through the development of advanced training for trainers.
- Providing mutual assistance and support in securing the legal basis for:
    - professional standards with regard to the ethical principles in exercising the profession;
    - recognition between countries of anthroposophically extended psychotherapy;
    - development of research goals within the meaning of the preamble.
- Assurance of professional ethical principles with regard to

patients, and mutual help and support for the members of the International Federation in their endeavour to promote

- the maintenance of professional ethical standards, both legally and spiritually;
- respect for our fellow human beings and respect for the freedom of the individual in body, soul and spirit.

Work in the School of Spiritual Science

The group for psychotherapy in the School of Spiritual Science at the Goetheanum has now existed for 20 years and meets in the context of the annual conference of the Medical Section. There are meanwhile about 50 colleagues who study the class lessons in greater depth.

For some years an initiative group from the department of internal medicine at the Filder Clinic has, on the basis of Rudolf Steiner's class lessons, worked on various topics in the anthroposophical understanding of the human being such as pathogenesis, trauma and psychiatric clinical pictures.

Both groups fundamentally work on the questions of our time from an esoteric perspective.

Publications

1. The German Society for Anthroposophic Psychotherapy/DTGAP has published an important first work. Johannes Reiner has edited and published the book *In der Nacht sind wir zwei Menschen* (At Night We Are Two People). Twenty-one authors have provided contributions and thus represent a good cross-section of what lives today in anthroposophic psychotherapy in Germany.[116] The title has been taken from a lecture by Rudolf Steiner. The central theme of the lecture cycle is the human being who can be grasped on the one hand materially and with the sense organs but on the other hand is non-sensory, i.e. spiritual. In the waking, conscious state these two spheres of existence are intermeshed and are one whereas in the darkness of night soul and spirit separate and the sleeping body lies in an unconscious state separated from sentience and memory.[117]

2. The Dutch book by Ad Dekkers about psychotherapeutic methodology was published in German by the German publisher Verlag Freies Geistesleben in September 2012: *Psychotherapie der menschlichen Würde* (Psychotherapy of Human Dignity). English, Italian and Spanish translations have been completed, a Russian one is in preparation. The content of the book is the result of 25 years of intercollegial and international studies, research through case studies and teaching the advanced training for anthroposophically-based psychotherapy. The latter started directly after Prof. B. C. J. Lievegoed had held his first and only advanced training for anthroposophically-based psychotherapy. The book was also written out of a concern that – apart from some good and beneficial psychotherapeutic endeavours – there is a trend in psychotherapy worldwide which increasingly aims for the monosymptomatic management of symptoms and short-term treatment by standardised protocols. On the other hand a tendency is spreading for short-term methodological relief of symptoms, while both tendencies are moving away from both a complex full picture of the human being and social, context-related pathogenesis. Both tendencies present themselves as evidence-based. The book aims to set itself in full in the context of historical and modern psychotherapy. Hence a number of professional authors are discussed.

3. Wolfgang Rissmann, Ad Dekkers and Janna Ertl have taken up the task of collecting fundamental passages on psychiatry in Rudolf Steiner's works. An article in this respect appeared in *Merkurstab*, volume 66, issue 3, May-June 2013, "Angaben zu Psychiatrie im Werk Rudolf Steiners". The 70 (!) individual references to questions of psychiatry are listed chronologically and there is a brief description of their content.

4. There is already an Italian translation of the book *Borderline Erkrankungen*, Verlag Freies Geistesleben, by Dieter Beck †, Ursula Langerhorst and Henriette Dekkers, with a foreword by Michaela Glöckler, under the title *Malattie Borderline*, Verlag Novalis, Milan 2005. In May 2011 a Spanish translation was published, translated by Dr med. Miguel Martínez Falero, general practitioner and psychotherapist, president of the anthroposophic medical association in Spain and of the "Betula" Association for Anthroposophic Psychotherapy. The book is called:

Trastorno Límite de Personalidad Borderline, Verlag Rudolf Steiner, Madrid. In August 2011, the Portuguese translation by Ralf Rickli was published by Ad Verbum – Anthroposófica on occasion of the foundation of the Brazilian anthroposophic psychotherapy association. The initiative and finance came from the professional group in Curitiba, Brazil.

5. In the USA Robert Sardello has published *Facing the World with Soul*, *Money and The Soul's Path of Virtue, Freeing the Soul from Fear:* all Lindisfarne Press.

William Bento has published a long list of books and articles on psychodiagnostics and psychotherapy. Worth mentioning are: Bento, W. (2004), *Lifting the Veil of Mental Illness: An Approach to Anthroposophical Psychology,* Great Barrington, MA: SteinerBooks (2009). *A Somatic Psycho-Diagnostic Approach to Personality Disorders*. Cologne, Germany: all Lambert Academic Publishing.

Post-graduate training

One of the main tasks of the IKAM coordinators was formulated as early as in the IKAM annual report of 2005: to answer the requests for anthroposophically-based psychotherapy by means of country-specific post-graduate training in accordance with agreed professional criteria and subsequently to encourage the establishment of national professional associations so that the work as a whole can be continued locally. This main task is now widely crystallising out.

Train the Trainers conference

In June 2014 a Train the Trainers conference took place for the first time, organised by certified colleagues from twelve countries. The goal is to draw up guidelines for a common, well-founded basis for teaching methodology, content and esoteric schooling.

A compendium of contributions from participants is in preparation to this end.

International Postgraduate Medical Training/IPMT

Anthroposophic psychotherapy spreads in two ways. On the one hand through a concrete enquiry from a country: a group of interested psychotherapists forms who organise further training for themselves and subsequent to the further training establish a society. The other way goes via the IPMTs. Here everyone in a country comes together who is interested in working with Anthroposophic Medicine and learning about it. All medical professional groups are represented. The group of psychotherapists then separate because they partly have their own programme. But the IPMT remains an important part of the further training. The advantages are clear: there is integration among the various professional groups from the beginning and the psychotherapists deepen their knowledge of Anthroposophic Medicine with regard to the physical foundations. Subsequently there is still a "certification week". This "IPMT model" is valid for Spanish-speaking South America and Asia. The IPMT model is currently operating for Chile, Argentina and India. Michaela Glöckler is the driving force because she is convinced that psychotherapy can give important and effective answers to the fragmentation problems of the modern human being and has its antenna extended throughout the world.

Research

For research itself there are not yet fully formulated goals. The ongoing projects relate to depression and attachment disorders as part of multidisciplinary treatment (Netherlands, together with the University of Applied Sciences Leiden) and the evaluation of interdisciplinary treatment for psychosomatic illness (Germany, Havelhöhe, M. Quetz).

Mantras for the psychotherapist

Psychotherapy has a fundamental meditation in the Young Physicians Course in the verse:

> "Push forward infancy into childhood ..."

This meditation brings the pre-birth aspect of the physical and etheric parts of the human being into intimate connection with the future aspect of the astral entity in great images. It serves to allow the psychotherapist to encompass the stream of coming-into-being and what has happened. The psychotherapists have this verse in common with those undertaking biography work.

Push forward infancy
Into childhood
And childhood
Into youth.
To you will appear condensed
Human etheric existence
Behind physical being –

Push back the density of old age
Into the period of human maturity
And maturity
Into youthful life.
To you will resound in cosmic tones
Human soul activity
Out of etheric life.

Rudolf Steiner[118]

A deepening of the understanding of the (psycho-)pathological dynamic can be brought about by the verse:

See in thy soul
    Power of radiance
Feel in thy body
    Might of heaviness
In the power of radiance
    Shines spirit-I
In the might of heaviness
    God's spirit works with strength
Yet shall not
    Power of radiance
Grasp

Might of heaviness
Nor
Might of heaviness
Penetrate
Power of radiance
For if power of radiance grasps
Might of heaviness
And if might of heaviness penetrates
Power of radiance
Soul and body
Will be bound to their ruin
In cosmic confusion.

Rudolf Steiner[119]

In the endeavour to understand the approach of physicians and priests and to demarcate their work from the professional group of psychotherapists, and in order to find the right place for the independence of consciousness between medication and sacrament, the meditation "I will go the path"[120] can provide orientation.

In psychotherapy this verse is additionally pondered by the astral body of the soul. It was made the foundation of the professional group for psychological psychotherapists and psychiatrists by Prof. Bernard Lievegoed. The verse is intended to place those working in medicine and psychotherapy into the mutually formed esoteric framework of the differentiated physical incarnation and to guide them upwards to the spiritualisation of these forces in order to lead to abilities of the soul. It is a verse which Rudolf Steiner gave to Ita Wegman:

I hold the sun within me
He guides me into the world as a king

I hold the moon within me
She retains my form

I hold Mercury within me
He holds the sun and moon together

I hold Venus within me
Without her love all things are nought

She with Mars unites herself
Who speaks my being in words

That Jupiter may enlighten all
With his wise light

And Saturn in maturity
In me lights up my being's colours

These are the seven of the world
I am the seven, across the earth
I am the world,
I am the sun.

(And Christian Rosenkreutz with cross and roses stands next to you as spirit)

I receive
The world
In the Seven.

Rudolf Steiner to Ita Wegman 1923/1924,
Notebook entry

Psychotherapists deal with the destiny of their patients. The closing sentences of this meditative verse are significantly deepening, they break through the outer appearance of happiness and pain and open up the karmic dimensions and lend the therapist unshakeable equilibrium:

Resting in future's lap:
"Anyone who believes that good fortune alone is beneficial,
bad things alone weigh us down, does not see
the year but only the day."

Rudolf Steiner[121]

Special needs education and social therapy
Basics – structures – perspectives

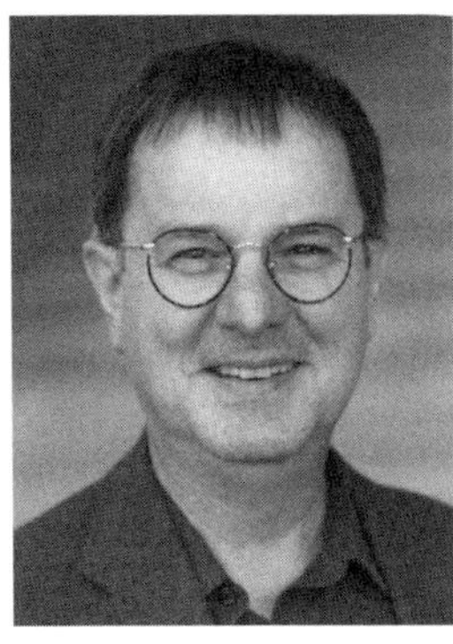

Prof. Dr Rüdiger Grimm, Dipl. Päd.,
Secretary
Council for Curative Education and Social Therapy
khs@khsdornach.org
www.khsdornach.org

Anthroposophical special needs education and social therapy

The range of tasks of special needs education and social therapy relates to helping, supporting, accompanying and treating children, young people and adults with developmental disorders and disabilities, with difficulties of learning and social interaction as well as supporting the processes of inclusion in social and societal life. Every special needs or social therapy measure or structure aims at the biographical development of the individuality of each person who make their way through life with their own opportunities and restrictions. The intention is to support its development in its respective environment. Institutional forms of special needs education and social therapy have the task of promoting the development of the individual and contributing to a successful life in inclusive social contexts.

Special needs education and social therapy are an interdisciplinary work field within which practically all professions working within the sphere of the Medical Section are active, as well as members of educational and social professions. Since the needs of people with disabilities can vary a great deal, a great variety of collaborative constellations may apply.

Physicians, including specialists, are as a rule the first people who come into contact with developmental problems in a child, diagnose them and initiate the first measures. They frequently undertake accompanying constitutional treatments and medical care if a disability is associated with a chronic illness. The work of therapists (eurythmy therapists, art therapists, physiotherapists, etc.) involves the treatment of special situations or problems.

Special needs teachers and kindergarten childcare workers support the development of children and young people in the processes of their upbringing and teach skills and abilities for future life. Special needs workers help in the medium of everyday life to initiate processes for successfully coping with life.

Social therapists and the associated professions have the task of helping adults needing support to lead a successful life with social inclusion in the spheres of work and culture.

Working with parents and relatives is of particular importance in all processes of special needs education and social therapy.

Beyond the work of the individual professions, special needs education and social therapy is a transdisciplinary work field which is most effective when more is created in the collaboration between the professions than is represented by the individual measures. Crucial for effective collaboration is that all those working together share a common basis of understanding which makes the so-called "child case meetings", special needs meetings or social therapeutic "biographical conversation" workable.

This basis can be found by way of example in the twelve lectures of the "Curative Education Course" which Rudolf Steiner gave in the summer of 1924 after the first practical initiatives for special needs education had been set up in three places – at the Waldorf School in Stuttgart, the Clinical and Therapeutic Institute in Arlesheim and the Therapeutic and Educational Institute for Children in Need of Special Care in Jena.

These lectures, which build on the anthroposophical understanding of the human being and the educational and medical systems developed by Steiner in the preceding years, contain basic ideas and approaches for special needs diagnosis and practice which contribute to a spiritual understanding of the human being and the associated psychosomatic processes of physical, emotional and spiritual development.

Beyond that, special needs education and social therapy are also genuinely social impulses. For the phenomena of disability are in their complexity almost always also associated with explicit or subtle processes of social exclusions. Thus anthroposophical special needs education and social therapy has also established places for a life together in which social life, work and culture is enabled for everyone.

Anthroposophical special needs education and social therapy are, however, not restricted to specific institutional forms but can bear fruit in all situations where we are concerned with the development, education and inclusion of people in need of support.

Structures of collaboration

It is the task of the Council for Curative Education and Social Therapy to build networks for the special needs education and social therapy work in meanwhile almost 50 countries with a total of more than 750 establishments and organisations and to ensure regular collaboration, exchange and reciprocal support. The paper "Basics and Method of Operation of the Council for Curative Education and Social Therapy" contains the agreements on the mode of such collaboration (www.khsdornach.org).

The countries – depending on the number of their establishments and organisations – appoint one or several representatives who participate in the annual closed conferences. The issues relevant at an international level are worked on there. More specialised issues of special needs education and social therapy are dealt with in the working groups set up for that purpose. Currently there are the following working groups:

- International Training Group with training council and approvals group
- Social therapy working group
- Physicians working in the field of special needs education and social therapy
- ECCE, European Co-operation in Anthroposophical Curative Education and Social Therapy

- Science group
- Economic group
- Coordination group

The Council for Curative Education and Social Therapy maintains a secretariat in Dornach which coordinates the international collaboration and represents the Council to the outside.

Services

The Council for Curative Education and Social Therapy organises an international conference for curative education and social therapy at the Goetheanum in Dornach every two years. In addition it organises various specialist conferences on academic and professional questions and subjects, as well as study days for members of the School of Spiritual Science working in the field of special needs education and social therapy. Its events are announced in the journal *Zeitschrift Seelenpflege* and on its website.

The Council undertakes its own research and development projects and works in an advisory capacity with other initiatives. Alongside publishing the specialist journal *Seelenpflege in Heilpädagogik und Sozialtherapie* it is also the publisher of the book series "Anthropos – Heilpädagogik und Sozialtherapie aus anthroposophischen Perspektiven" which has appeared since 2012 in cooperation with the publishers Verlag am Goetheanum and Athena Verlag as well as other publishing projects.

In its academic work and the development of academic training opportunities, it works together with Alanus University of Arts and Social Sciences in Alfter.

The Council has an up-to-date online bibliography of literature on anthroposophical special needs education and social therapy as well as a reference library of the existing literature. It publishes a directory of all establishments for special needs education and social therapy working from an anthroposophical perspective.

A central work area is the collaboration with national organisations, relatives' and professional associations and with special needs education and social therapy establishments worldwide.

Training and further training

Training and further training are future capital. The development of anthroposophical methods for working with people with disabilities is dependent on young people being able to find high quality training opportunities in which they can study the foundations of special needs education and social therapy in the anthroposophical understanding of the human being. The latter must at the same time be associated with full professional training, i.e. as a rule state recognition. Currently there are training opportunities both at the college and university level. The anthroposophical training centres have combined to form an international training group in which they can work on specialist aspects, issues of quality development and advanced training projects.

Economic basis

The Council for Curative Education and Social Therapy has its own legal entity in the "Fonds für Heilpädagogik und Sozialtherapie" (a so-called non-registered association under Swiss law). It receives its funding primarily in the form of contributions from the countries working together in the Council as well as from income from publications and donations. Projects are each financed through their own project budget for which third party funding is, as a rule, raised. The Council's annual report is published in issue 2 of *Zeitschrift Seelenpflege* in the following year and on the website of the Council.

Perspectives

Special needs and social therapy provisions are fundamentally public, they can be used by everyone and in many countries are part of the social support systems. As such they are both actors in the societal transformation processes and affected by the changing framework conditions for social work. Thus they face the challenge to make their own specific contribution to public discourse.

In order to represent this contribution convincingly, the

further academic development of the foundations of anthroposophical special needs education and social therapy which has been initiated must be rigorously pursued. The image of the human being of anthroposophy and the social forms of special needs education and social therapy which have for many years been given practical expression represent an important foundation for the development of inclusive provisions for people with disabilities; but their institutional forms will have to change in the foreseeable future in order to continue with innovation in society.

A series of establishments have already developed interesting and forward-looking provisions in this respect. For others it will not be easy to jettison ballast and keep up with the latest developments. In not a few others it is indeed a question whether and to what extent they wish to continue to be associated with the methods and foundations of anthroposophical special needs education and social therapy.

In an international context it could be observed that not all hopeful initiatives were able to maintain and develop themselves in the political and economic developments of their countries – some of them also because of internal problems of their own. Not a few of them have, however, undertaken innovative and resilient work under the most adverse of circumstances, particularly where they have managed to mobilise their own social circle.

It might even happen that the number of anthroposophical establishments will fall. But our movement has from the beginning defined itself first and foremost by quality and to a certain extend also reflected critically on the quantitative aspect. The international development of anthroposophical special needs education and social therapy continues apace: thus in the past few years there has been a growing awareness of anthroposophy and its impulses for practical social life in the Asia-Pacific region and thus a demand for the development of provisions for people with special developmental needs.

Information at www.khsdornach.org with current conferences and publications, the structural papers of the international "Council Network" and the Council's annual reports.

Spiritual foundations of special needs education and social therapy

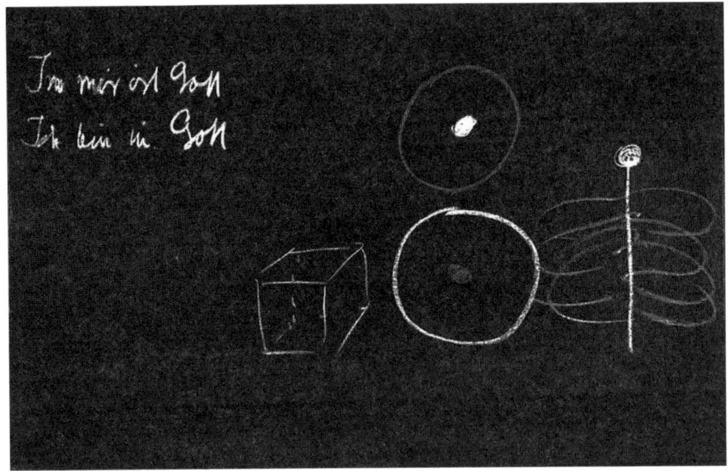

Blackboard drawing by Rudolf Steiner for the "point and circle meditation"

Rudolf Steiner's Curative Education Course contains a series of meditative exercises for deepening the questions and problems related to special needs education and the anthroposophical understanding of the human being so that they become an inner and own experience.[122] We can see the point and circle meditation (see above) as being at the centre of these exercises; it was not given by Rudolf Steiner until towards the end of the course in lectures 10 and 11.

It is an exercise which enables us meditatively to experience the fundamental, polar relationships between the forces which act in the human organisation, e.g. for instance in the contrasting images of the compulsive reproduction of always the same ideas on the one hand and the inability to remember even the most simple everyday experiences on the other. The understanding of and work in special needs education thus arise from a process of convergence between external observation, insight into the anthroposophical understanding of the human being, the inner recreating and envisaging of constitutional processes, as well as the establishment of an empathetic relationship with and the development of individual provisions for people in need of special care.

The point and circle meditation

The inner activity involved in the point and circle meditation encompasses several elements by means of which polar experiences can be stimulated and deepened:

Practicing it in the evening and morning means that it engages with differing states of consciousness: in the evening a contemplative awareness arises as we recall the past day and release ourselves from its events and experiences – which can now be formed into inner pictures in retrospective review. In the morning, on the other hand, we enter the individual space of our actions which we are likely to envisage in thoughts in a goal-oriented way, but which in principle is open for what may result, and is co-determined by what comes to meet it. The polar situation in which we live can be experienced meditatively at the transitions between sleeping and waking.

A second polar element is practiced through the formal dynamic of point and circle, that is to say through the inner exercise of forming images of centripetal and centrifugal movement. In our mind's eye the point undergoes a movement that continually expands towards the circle, while at the same time the peripheral circle element increasingly concentrates towards the point.

The associated use of blue and yellow likewise points to the greatest possible contrast of colour spaces – of space-creating and receding impressions on the one hand, and emerging and luminous ones on the other.

The two short meditative phrases enable us to live our way into the depth of these processes: to experience the activity that gives rise to consciousness in the evening not just as a reflection of day consciousness but as the presence of a spiritual reality in which divine thoughts can fill human awareness: "God is in me". In morning consciousness, on the other hand, we can experience how, in acting, our will activity touches and affects not only a world of objects but at the same time also a divinely created world in which we encounter each other with our individual destinies and dispositions: "I am in God".

Inner flexibility can arise from ongoing practice of this meditation, harmonising the transitions between states of consciousness in human beings of waking thinking and sleeping will. As a "professional meditation" it enables us to acquire experiences which are ultimately indispensable for work in special needs education: it is a schooling of mindfulness, of reverence for the world of the senses and its often unexpected pointers and key opportunities for perceiving another being. And it creates a developmental space for the confidence to be able to act in the moment with presence of mind.

Special needs education and social therapy as a profession?

Pleasure in the encounter with other people, interest in the human organisation, support of physical, emotional and cognitive difficulties, creation of a developmental and living environment as well as building bridges to societal and social life form the core of the professions in special needs education and social therapy. Practical work and reflection on goals and actions form an indivisible unit, as does the question how to deal with our own shortcomings and experiences of confrontation – an exciting and challenging profession. It provides the opportunity for attentiveness towards others, for consciously dealing with ourselves and a proactive attitude with regard to social and cultural processes.

Eurythmy therapy

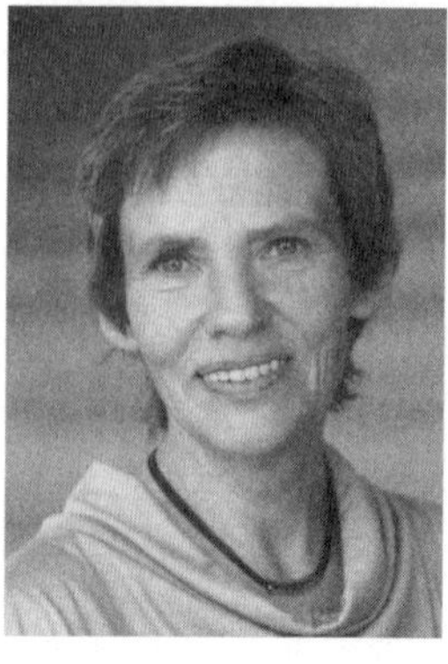

Angelika Jaschke, eurythmy therapist
International Coordination of Eurythmy Therapy
ajaschke@heileurythmie-medsektion.net
http://heileurythmie-medsektion.net

What is the position of eurythmy therapy in the system of Anthroposophic Medicine?

Eurythmy therapy is the only profession in the system of Anthroposophic Medicine which exclusively comes from Rudolf Steiner's spiritual science and has its foundation in it. The professional community of eurythmy therapists has continued to develop since 2000 out of needs and necessities in the International Eurythmy Therapy Forum through a common global awareness.

Meanwhile approximately 1,600 eurythmy therapists are working in more than 40 countries under a great variety of different conditions to make the eurythmy therapy impulse within the anthroposophic medical movement accessible for patients. In this way a flexible organism has been created which is guided both by the societal requirements and the inner, spiritual questions.

How is the association of eurythmy therapists organised? How is it financed?

Expert panels work autonomously on specific subject areas. There is a coordinator from each expert panel, a person who has set themselves the task of having an overview over the whole network in order thereby to motivate further developmental steps in the specific expert panel. These coordinators together form the so-called coordinator team.

There are currently the following expert panels:

1. Representatives from all **training courses** recognised by the Medical Section at the Goetheanum (about 10 worldwide) work together in the international trainer conference (GbR) on questions of training quality, the method and with regard to recognition under the regulations governing the professions. The agreements reached mutually in this group are binding for "recognition by the Medical Section".
2. A **research** colloquium among active researchers promotes the exchange of views and works on a specific eurythmy therapy research concept – in collaboration with the existing AM research institutes.
3. **Thirteen professional associations** have combined worldwide with regard to legal questions and cooperations as well as quality development (AnthroMed®) going beyond national concerns (IAg-HEBV). A legal **federation** with the associations for eurythmy therapy and anthroposophical art therapies (IFAAET) is concerned with European and international legal issues and is actively involved in expanding the system of AM.
4. Deepening work is undertaken in the existing **six practice fields** (work with small children, school children, people with special needs, patients in hospital, the elderly and in independent practice) through further training and work on the understanding of the human being at various ages in the context of eurythmy therapy.
5. Public relations work is supported through a **website** with all basic standards for eurythmy therapy, information, addresses and links, an internal specialist discussion forum as well as publications. www. heileurythmie-medsektion.net.
6. The Eurythmy Therapy Forum is **financed** through a voluntary solidarity contribution from all international eurythmy therapists to the value of one national hour of therapy per year. This raises about half of what is needed to cover the necessary costs. Sponsors, legacies and foundations finance projects as far as possible.

How are the modes of work and responsibility structures described in this book practiced in eurythmy therapy?

At the annual delegate conference (responsible representatives from training, research, professional associations, countries, practice fields, study in the First Class of the School of Spiritual Science, public relations and other work contexts) there is an international exchange of views and pending questions are worked on. The work that needs to be done is organised and responsibility is taken for it by individual people in mutual recognition and growing trust.

Feedback to the national, decentralised persons responsible and individuals with whom the task of decision-making and implementation lies, takes place through the delegates.

This path requires the willingness to take on joint responsibility for the current and future tasks of eurythmy therapy and to know and want to keep oneself spiritually connected. It is like a heart organ in which the periphery and centre are in constant dynamically fluid exchange and fertilise one another.

The expert panels, the coordination team and the IKAM coordinator take on the responsibility for the worldwide development of eurythmy therapy within the anthroposophic medical movement. This includes both work on specialist and professional development through training and advanced training (further training is subject to the regulations of the national professional associations), the agreement of standards for the reciprocal recognition of training qualifications, consultancy in specialist and professional policy questions, the development of relations with other professional and task fields in the Medical Section as well as the cultivation of work on the esotericism of the profession and involvement in the First Class of the School of Spiritual Science.

How is training organised and where is information available?

The international trainers' conference is the oldest body in the eurythmy therapy. It has met since 1983 with the joint responsibility of developing the methodological and practical foundations of the training courses in joint work – guided by the questions of the world as it is at present.

Reciprocal recognition as the expression of collaboration based on equal status and commitment is an important process for quality development and identity formation internally and externally. The basic requirements for the content of eurythmy therapy training are laid down in the "International Framework Curriculum" and this continues to be worked on as necessary. The procedure developed in the accreditation handbook of the Medical Section is used by most of the training courses. An important part of this quality procedure is, among other things, the audit across professions as a help for self-reflection and self-correction.

Most training courses today are part-time. All of them – in accordance with the "International Framework Curriculum" currently in force – build on a basic eurythmy training leading to a diploma or Bachelor. There are currently seven ongoing training courses worldwide and three to four training courses in various countries which undertake a single two- or three-year course under the sponsorship of a recognised training course. Further information at: http://www.heileurythmie-medsektion.net/de/tr/ausbildung.

How is the spiritual substance cultivated?

Rudolf Steiner spoke the following words in Munich on 28 August 1913 when the members of the Anthroposophical Society were shown EURYTHMY for the first time: "*But observe also that a threefold will underlies this eurythmy.*"

He characterised the three elements of this underlying will on 15 May 1920

- as *the aesthetic, the element of beauty*. Intensified movements of the higher worlds are an artistic element: "*In the art of eurythmy human beings themselves are the instrument.*"
- as the *educational and teaching element*. Here the task is to connect the human soul with the physical body in such a way that the soul can develop and unfold. As elsewhere, on 15 May 1920 educational eurythmy is also called "*ensouled gymnastics*".

- as the *hygienic and therapeutic element*. That is to say, becoming attentive to *"what the etheric body, through its inner flexibility, really requires of the physical body"*, and overcoming the disharmony between physical and etheric body through a *"capacity of movement of the physical body that corresponds to the etheric body – harmony with cosmic being"*.

The only meditation specifically given for eurythmy is based on this archetypal will nature that underlies all forms of eurythmy (art, education and therapy).[123] It is in connection with the living, human eurythmical instrument of the body, the soul and the spiritual-cosmic surroundings – that is, the whole human being – that the forces at work in it, the effective actions and also the physical loci of manifestation are named. The spiritual space resounds through *"earth – air – heaven"*, soul activity through *"speech – singing – thinking"*, and the physical form through *"feet – hands – head"*.

"In the case of eurythmists too, it can only be a matter of rendering themselves receptive to sensing and feeling expressive gestures by repeatedly awakening a certain mood of soul. Then, through a meditation that penetrates to the secrets of the human organisation, the eurythmist can enter into this subtle sensing. This can be achieved, for instance, by meditating on the words with full inwardness, with strong, inner sensing of their content – so that what you meditate on does not remain mere words or abstract concepts but that what the words contain really is accomplished in you; then you will achieve what I have just described.

I seek within
The working of creative forces,
The life of creative powers.
Earth's gravity
Is telling me
Through the word of my feet,
Air's power of form
Is telling me
Through the singing of my hands,

Heaven's strength of light
Is telling me
Through the thinking of my head
How the world in human beings
Speaks, sings, contemplates.

Once you have done such a meditation, you will find you can say about yourself that you have as if awoken from cosmic sleep into the heavenly quality of eurythmy. When you wake up from night into day, you will always enter into the quality of eurythmy if you awaken this mood within you" (author's italics).[124]

- - -

In eurythmy we are further familiar with six eurythmical form meditations which we can describe as an "esoteric resource" and which, properly practised, are meditative in character. Since of first World Eurythmy Therapy Conference in 2008, the impulse adopted there is alive that each eurythmy therapist at the start of their therapeutic day performs a/their eurythmical meditation in the awareness of the whole professional community worldwide. Thus a world-enveloping eurythmical meditative movement goes around the world each day with the course of the sun. This has meanwhile become an etheric envelope which is a real experience.

These are exercises which in their archetypal form are carried out in standing:

IAO
SM-HM
Five-pointed star (steadfast I stand)
Light streams upwards, weight bears downwards
I think speech
Halleluja
TAO

In his course on tone eurythmy Rudolf Steiner says: "*Then you will see that in the TAO you have a wonderful resource for making your inner corporeality supple, inwardly flexible and artisti-*

cally amenable for eurythmy ... You will find when you do this that it gives you inner strength which you can transpose to all eurythmy. This is an esoteric resource. And to do this means meditation in eurythmy" (author's italics).[125]

As part of his lectures about the Rosicrucian principles of alchemy, Rudolf Steiner in a different context speaks about the way in which the forces of the upper organisation (light) and the lower one (heaviness) are symbolically represented in two triangles which, although they interpenetrate one another, do not mix. We are familiar with this as one of the six form meditations in eurythmy: "*Light streams upwards, weight bears downwards*".[126]

The last meditation of the Christmas course for young physicians is about the daily battle between sickness and health, between matter with its "might of heaviness" and the spirit with its "power of radiance": this meditation leads us to an understanding of a process within the human being.

"Now, to think all these things with the necessary moral impulse, to penetrate them with feeling, to sense them fully, and then to imbue what you have felt with will, enables you to gradually learn to observe things, the world's processes, in the following way: that, when radiance has grasped hold of the might of heaviness, you separate this radiance from the might of heaviness by means of something that supports the etheric body via the astral body through an outer substance, or through a process unfolding within the human being. You see, if you properly feel such a thing in your soul, you will also acquire a capacity to observe how eurythmy therapy heals. For the healing effect of eurythmy therapy is basically what I might describe as the thing which counts quite especially on cosmic forces. If you do the consonantal eurythmy therapy exercises, you are embedded in moon forces.

When you develop vowel forces in eurythmy therapy, then you are embedded in Saturn forces. And through these two types of forces human beings feel their way directly into the cosmos when they practice eurythmy therapy" (author's italics).[127]

See in thy soul
    Power of radiance
Feel in thy body
    Might of heaviness
In the power of radiance
    Shines spirit-I
In the might of heaviness
    God's spirit works with strength
Yet shall not
    Power of radiance
Grasp
    Might of heaviness
Nor
    Might of heaviness
Penetrate
    Power of radiance
For if power of radiance grasps
    Might of heaviness
And if might of heaviness penetrates
    Power of radiance
Soul and body
    Will be bound to their ruin
In cosmic confusion.

Rudolf Steiner[128]

Rudolf Steiner states that a general need for healing in modern people is to regain a spiritual worldview that can overcome materialism. Only in this way can karmic conflicts from previous incarnations be morally resolved rather than somatising themselves as illness.

The first meditation in the Easter course for young physicians calls on us to see the whole development of the human being within the cosmos as it now is.[129]

Only the physical body itself belongs to the earth and is attracted by it. The etheric body works entirely out of the cosmos, forming the physical body with its peripheral forces of suction.

Today it is forgotten "that the human form must certainly be derived from what gives us knowledge of the starry heavens, but in an inner, qualitative sense" (author's italics).[130]

If we wish to understand the human being, "[...] we have to look out into the universal cosmos".[131]

Behold, what is joined in the cosmos,
Thou feelest the forming of the human being.

Behold, all that moves thee in air,
Thou wilt experience the human being's ensoulment.

Behold, what is changed in the earthly,
Thou wilt discern the spiritualising of the human being.[132]

This meditation given to the young physicians has an inner connection with the profoundest concern of eurythmy therapy – understood as an earthly-cosmic medicine.

Only through our ongoing effort to connect each sound repeatedly anew with the zodiacal and planetary forces can the healing effect of eurythmy therapy be revealed in full.

- - -

And last but not least, let us refer here to the Foundation Stone meditation which Rudolf Steiner "entrusted" to all members of the Anthroposophical Society for cultivating and healing the spiritual community building within it.

Human soul!
You live in the limbs
Which carry you through the world of space
Into the ocean of spirit being:
Practise spirit recall
In depths of soul,
Where in the reign
Of cosmic creator existence
Your own I
In God's I
Is begotten;

And you will truly live
In human cosmic being.

Because the Father spirit rules on high
Creating being in the cosmic depths:
You spirits of power,
Let from the heights resound
What in the depths is echoed;
Speaking:
Of the divine is humanity born.
It is heard by spirits in east, west, north, south:
Let human beings hear it.

Human soul!
You live in the beat of heart and lung,
Which leads you through the rhythm of time
Into the feeling of your own soul's being:
Practice spirit contemplation
In equilibrium of soul,
Where the surging cosmic creative deeds
Unite
Your own I
With the cosmic I;
And you will truly feel
In human soul's creating.

For Christ's will rules in the surrounding sphere
Granting grace to souls in cosmic rhythms:
You spirits of light,
Let from the east ignite
What through the west is formed.
Speaking:
In Christ death turns into life.
It is heard by spirits in east, west, north, south:
Let human beings hear it.

Human soul!
You live in the resting head,
Which from the bedrock of eternity

Opens cosmic thoughts:
Practice spirit beholding
In the stillness of thoughts,
Where the eternal goals of gods
Bestow
Cosmic being's light
On your own I
For your free willing;
And you will truly think
In depths of human spirit.

For the spirit's cosmic thoughts reign
In cosmic being, light imploring:
You spirits of soul,
Let from the depths request
What will be heard in the heights:
Speaking:
The soul awakens in spirit's cosmic thoughts.
It is heard by spirits in east, west, north, south:
Let human beings hear it.

At the turning point of time
The cosmic spirit light entered
The stream of earth existence;
Night's rule of darkness
Had come to an end;
The bright light of day
Shone brightly in human souls;
Light,
That gives warmth
To poor shepherds' hearts;
Light,
That enlightens
The wise heads of kings.

Divine light,
Sun of Christ
Warm
Our hearts;

Enlighten
Our heads;
That good may become,
What from
Our hearts we found,
What from
Our heads
We want to guide with purpose.

Rudolf Steiner[133]

Anthroposophic art therapy

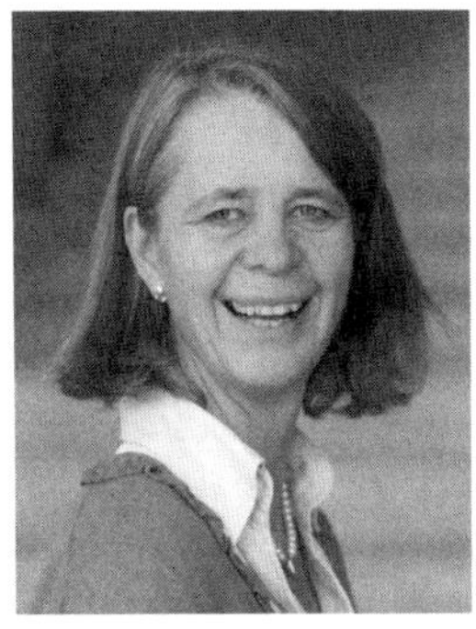

Kirstin Kaiser, therapeutic creative speech practitioner and art therapist ED
International Coordination of Art Therapy
kirstinkaiser@bluewin.ch
www.icaat-medsektion.net
www.medsektion-goetheanum.org

What is the contribution of anthroposophic art therapy in the system of Anthroposophic Medicine?

The laws acting in the imbalances of illness in human beings can also be found in the arts. Colours, forms, tones and sounds are newly created and recreated into works of art in therapy and influence body, soul and spirit. In artistic activity patients can intervene in the disease processes in a creative and transformative way. Encouraging and supporting such an active path of conscious work on our own destiny is the therapeutic task. In this context each art form makes its own differentiated contribution in terms of the anthroposophical understanding of the human being. Approximately 1,500 anthroposophical art therapists work worldwide.

Training and further training in anthroposophic art therapy

Anthroposophic art therapists are trained in state-recognised colleges and in training courses and further training courses under private law which lead to professional qualifications.

Recognition as an anthroposophic art therapist by the Medical Section is preceded by an approval process.

How is the International Coordination of Art Therapy organised?

The coordination field of "Anthroposophic art therapy" is represented by an art therapist who works in close contact with various bodies working in the field and who is affirmed by the latter in his or her task. These bodies exist for the areas: professional associations, training, conference organisation, public relations work, research and representation in IKAM. There are representatives for the specialist fields of painting, modelling, music and "therapeutic creative speech" who are responsible for coordinating their field. The organogram with the names of the contacts can be found on the website www.icaat-MedSection.net.

The executive councils of the national professional associations (DAKART) meet twice a year for an intensive exchange of views. Thus an international occupational profile and ethics guidelines were drawn up for example. Once a year the representatives of the professional associations meet with the members of the European Academy for Anthroposophical Art Therapy to align training and professional associations. In September 2012, the International Federation of Anthroposophic Arts and Eurythmy Therapy (IFAAET) was established together with the executive council members for eurythmy therapy. The purpose of this community is

- to represent the national anthroposophic art therapy and eurythmy therapy associations at an international level.
- to support the development of anthroposophic art therapies and eurythmy therapy in countries in which there is no professional association and there is no reciprocal assistance and support.

- the further development of the international foundations of anthroposophic art therapies and eurythmy therapy under public law together with the Medical Section.

Conferences

International study days on anthroposophic art therapy and a study conference for creative speech take place annually at the Goetheanum in Dornach / Switzerland. The working groups are led collaboratively by an art therapist and a physician and thus enable the interdisciplinary exchange of views. The conference lectures are compiled and published.

Public relations work

There is information about the coordination work, training centres, professional associations, literature and much else on the website www.icaat-medsektion.net.

In addition, books on anthroposophical art therapy are being reissued, conference documentation published, and posters and flyers on art therapies and specific indications prepared.

Furthermore, work is taking place on a three-volume overview of all statements by Rudolf Steiner on the medical understanding of the human being relating to language. The first volume with search results and content is available as print-on-demand. The second volume will contain all relevant original quotes as source material. The third volume will contain a synopsis of these statements.

Academic research

The art therapies must set out their effectiveness, state of research and positioning within the medical guidelines. Here the broad background of experience of individual therapeutic measures is not enough; on the contrary, the academic evidence is crucial for funders. Hence only the art therapies with evidence-based documentation of their efficacy and effect will in the medium term be able to play a relevant role in the medical system!

There have not so far been sufficient resources to meet the

requirements of systematic evidence at an academic level. It is therefore an urgent objective at this time to create new structural, staff and financial facilities which can do justice to the requirements.

Protection of proprietary rights

Anthroposophic art therapists will in future be able to obtain certification in accordance with the AnthroMed® label quality criteria.

Finances

The Coordination of Anthroposophic Art Therapy is financed by the Medical Section, individual contributions from art therapists, contributions from national associations and training centres, and income from certification and accreditation. Project financing is through donations. The aim is for the coordination office to be financed from contributions from the art therapists. Without voluntary work in coordinating the training and professional associations, and in research and conference preparation, the Coordination would hardly be able to function.

How is the next generation supported in anthroposophic art therapy? What training, further training and advanced training provisions are there?

Training and advanced training in art therapy is divided into three areas: state-recognised colleges, training courses under private law providing a professional qualification, and advanced training.

a) Three state-recognised colleges in Germany and Holland which offer courses in anthroposophic art therapy have come together in a working group (Anthroposophic Art Therapy in Colleges with State Recognition, AKHsA) in order to collaborate with regard to teaching content for anthroposophic art therapy, questions of professional approval, and joint research projects. Some colleges are members of the European Academy.

b) The European Academy for Anthroposophic Art Therapies

(EA) is a grouping of training courses and colleges under private law which has taken on accreditation for training courses and advanced training courses for "Anthroposophic art therapists" within the Medical Section. The training directors of the member schools meet twice a year to work together on development issues and optimise and carry out the accreditation process.

Once the accreditation process was coordinated on an interdisciplinary basis within the framework of the Medical Section, audits are carried out by a trained interdisciplinary team of auditors.

An international conference of training directors takes place once a year at the Goetheanum.

How is spiritual substance cultivated in anthroposophic art therapy?

The approach to meditation in the field of anthroposophic art therapy is lived in very individual ways. Some examples of such paths will therefore be set out here. The meditation "See in thy Soul" inspires many colleagues by deepening the insight into the interplay of the forces of matter/might of heaviness and spirit/power of radiance. Meditative engagement with the nature of art and artistic means is one that we seek to practice consciously each day, supported by meditative texts by Rudolf Steiner which he gave for the various art forms.

Thoughts on the verse by Rudolf Steiner "See in thy Soul" from the perspective of therapeutic speech formation

Dietrich von Bonin

See in thy soul
    Power of radiance
Feel in thy body
    Might of heaviness
In the power of radiance

Shines spirit-I
In the might of heaviness
God's spirit works with strength
Yet shall not
Power of radiance
Grasp
Might of heaviness
Nor
Might of heaviness
Penetrate
Power of radiance
For if power of radiance grasps
Might of heaviness
And if might of heaviness penetrates
Power of radiance
Soul and body
Will be bound to their ruin
In cosmic confusion.

Rudolf Steiner[134]

(Translator's note: this article refers to the rhythms of the German original.) The verse contains three four-line stanzas. The first stanza is in trochaic metre (-v-). The two terms "Power of radiance" ("Leuchtekraft") and "Might of heaviness" ("Schweremacht") are each given a subsidiary, indented line of their own and, taken on their own, both assume an amphimacer meter (-v-) which is accentuated in inward, meditative speaking. The two last lines of the stanza are kept precisely symmetrical in the main line and indented line.

The second stanza introduces a radical change from falling to the rising rhythm of iambic meter (v-) which will carry us to the end of the verse (except in the very last line). Main and indented lines are constructed in a polar opposite meter: "Yet shall not" ("Doch darf nicht", v-v) / "Power of radiance" ("Leuchtekraft", -v-). Our rhythmic sensibility – corresponding with the admonishing content – feels itself awoken through this opposition.

The iambic meter continues in the last stanza. The first two lines lead with a certain inexorability, through their division of three metric feet in the main line and two feet in the subsidiary line, to the culmination formulated in the subsequent last lines: "For if power of radiance grasps / Might of heaviness" ("Denn fasset Leuchtekraft / die Schweremacht", v-v-v- / v-v-). Here in the last two lines, the previously clear rhythmical and metrical stream of inner will is as though shaken up by metrical irregularity – thus also conveying tumult and confusion "cosmic confusion" ("Welten-Irre") through the meter itself.

When we work with the meditation, speaking it externally and subsequently internally develops an intense feeling and will relationship with the text through its meter and rhythm. Further questions and discoveries follow: two worlds must be kept separate from each other. The one should be perceived, the other felt. Our therapeutic consciousness may initially miss a third, mediating entity here. But the riddle is resolved by the fact that rhythm embodies the free connection between temporal poles. Only between clearly separated opposites can mediating resonance arise, to form interest as the continually reborn rhythmic centre. Every excessive encroachment of one direction over the other ("grasps"/"fasset", "penetrates"/"dringet") immediately disrupts the rhythm.

To be in accord with the cosmos, our relationship to our body should become one of feeling, and our relationship to our own soul one of inner vision. Here the experiential question arises as to whether this relationship to our own being also applies to our therapeutic stance towards the patient, or whether different laws apply there. Surely it is the task of a therapist to behold the might of heaviness in the other and to illuminate it with the radiance of diagnostic insight. If the therapist were to feel the might of heaviness in the patient, this would be tantamount to an unjustified violation of boundaries.

Must we not likewise develop empathic feeling for the soul and spirit of the other and in this way give active forces of love. If, as therapists, we confine ourselves to diagnostic observation of the other's soul and spirit, those seeking help may easily experience themselves as being "professionally disregarded".

Thus, the gestures embodied in the two promptings, "see" ("schau") and "feel" ("fühl") seem to be directed, in relation to the patient, to the opposite aspect of their being. For the therapeutic speech practitioner, language is embodied in sounds which once formed the human body through the forces of the Logos, and which in speaking liberate themselves from it in order to be available to their bearer as a body for speech. To these sounds, to the body of speech, we should gain a feeling relationship, as Rudolf Steiner shows in exemplary fashion in his instructions for the first five articulation exercises: "Learn to feel every sound, become aware of your speech instruments."

On the other hand, the text's content also comes to meet us with luminous force engendered by the poet's individual soul and spirit. In the realm of language this corresponds to the soul's "power of radiance" ("Leuchtekraft"). To gain vision of this individual content will place us in the right relationship to it and enable us in recitation to give it a form that corresponds to its intrinsic nature. If, on the other hand, we feel the content of the text too personally, as naturally occurs at an initial stage of appropriation, then recitation – particularly conveying content to the patient – can be obscured by personal enjoyment or rejection, creating confusion.

Meditative practice with verses given by Rudolf Steiner for creative speech

Dietmar Ziegler

You find yourself:
Seeking in cosmic reaches,
Striving for cosmic heights.
Fighting in cosmic depths.

Rudolf Steiner[135]

(Translator's note: the comments in this article refer to the text in the German original.) In this verse, given as a breathing exercise, the I is taken hold of in feeling, thinking and the will through the three speech formulations.

According to Rudolf Steiner, it should be practised in such a way that the vowels and consonant clusters are deeply entered into and the flow of the breath gradually carries the speech outside in the air. Reason is initially only used cleverly to keep it out, i.e. it must overcome itself.

Three spheres of encounter between the I and the world are indicated and a specific soul activity is called up for each of them.

Seeking in the surroundings of the world: each encounter with a person or a something requires openness, willingness, dedication to the other if it is to bear fruit for the goal of this path: that the I grows into the soul body.

Striving with the power of enthusiasm to the heights of cosmic thoughts, like an eagle to the light, the free formative life force requires courage which, left completely to its own resources, must not become timid. The I is then strengthened in order, **fighting** and struggling for the human being, to become active in the physical world.

In terms of the language, the first sentence should be spoken with effect, but out of mature inner strength. The two short syllables, each beginning with D ("Du findest Dich selbst" – "You find yourself"), help in this respect. The colon at the end raises anticipation. Then a switch in the breathing before the second line; the soul streams out in the vowels, expanding into the surroundings, the consonants merely support it without interfering. Four differentiated E sounds at the end of the line help us to feel the encounter with the world ("Suchend in Weltenfernen" – "Seeking in cosmic reaches"). The letting go before the third line is important. Now the breathing extends itself and reaches upwards, concentrated and powerful in the consonant; the vowels become luminous and composed ("Strebend nach Weltenhöhen" – "Striving for cosmic heights").

Thereafter a moment of quiet is required in order consciously to inhale the depths. The last line goes wholly into rounding and bending the consonants with the warmth of the will because through the deeds of love the I becomes reality ("Kämpfend in Weltentiefen" – "Fighting in cosmic depths").

The meditative practice of painting therapy

Anita Kapfhammer, Rico Queisser

In the darkness I find God's being
2
In rose-red I feel the fount of life
3
In ether-blue rests spirit longing
4
In living green all things breathe breath of life
5
In golden yellow shines the clarity of thinking
6
In fiery red is rooted strength of will
7
In white of sun reveals itself my being's core.

Rudolf Steiner[136]

This verse by Rudolf Steiner can be spoken at the beginning of painting therapy work, at the start of each therapy session. Patients, too, feel themselves addressed by this colour meditation and always find a connection with themselves. The colour verse leaves us very free, and yet highly focused. It builds a wonderful bridge between everyday life and the world of colours which opens up. The verse leads to an experience of the nature of the colours themselves. The colour is already active as medicine in the words, and this is further intensified in colour preparation/mixing and above all in the painting process itself.

We know from Rudolf Steiner that colour is the soul of nature and of the whole cosmos, and that through our I which lives in the soul we raise ourselves from this fluctuating, burgeoning sea of colour and can thus form our soul into a consciousness soul. Through a path of schooling in painting (every art therapy is also a path of schooling) the soul undergoes, in the highest sense, a cultivation and purification so as to freely serve the human I and increasingly grasp hold of the etheric and physical organism in an ordering, formative way.

Painting in artistic striving is in itself meditation in the meaning of Schiller.[137] But as a meditative immersion in painting therapy, there is the colour meditation as developed by Rose Maria Pütz.[138] This method, which was developed for therapeutic use, serves equally well as a schooling path. By means of a highly diluted water or plant colour – which is developed in several layers of lazure in painting – and an atmosphere of calm and concentration, there can be a profound reflection on the colour. With an open-minded attitude, a sustained resonance with the respective nature of the colour can thus be produced through perception and inner listening, leading to greater insight and schooling us to open ourselves and increase our sensibility.

Meditations for anthroposophic music therapy

Viola Heckel and Marlise Maurer

Access to Rudolf Steiner's verse "See in thy Soul / Power of Radiance" from the perspective of the anthroposophic music therapist

See in thy soul
    Power of radiance
Feel in thy body
    Might of heaviness
In the power of radiance
    Shines spirit-I
In the might of heaviness
    God's spirit works with streng
Yet shall not
    Power of radiance
Grasp
    Might of heaviness
Nor
    Might of heaviness
Penetrate
    Power of radiance
For if power of radiance grasps
    Might of heaviness

And if might of heaviness penetrates
    Power of radiance
Soul and body
    Will be bound to their ruin
In cosmic confusion.

Rudolf Steiner[139]

If I direct my attention to the rhythmic resonance of the words of the meditation, I become aware of a dynamic which corresponds with its content: the swing of the pendulum between power of radiance and might of heaviness speeds up with the consequence that our experience is enhanced which expresses the danger of these two forces penetrating one another. The rhythmic quality at the level of the musicality of speech enables the verse not only to reach our rational mind but also allows us to develop an understanding that is sustained by the feeling level.

In swinging both to power of radiance and might of heaviness, my inner activity moves in opposite directions through a middle which continuously has to be acquired anew. This middle has the character of an interval. In music, the inaudible interval calls forth the actual musical experience which is described by Rudolf Steiner as a purely etheric experience. "The music becomes all the more ensouled the more you can bring to bear the inaudible part it contains."[140]

Power of radiance and might of heaviness are also revealed in the process of tone production. A tone touches us all the more, the more strongly it is illuminated by the soul's radiance. At the same time each tone must be well anchored in the body, strengthened by the might of heaviness. The meditation awakens a deeper understanding of the interplay between soul and body, between upper and lower organisation.

Sound meditation in music therapy

A unique form of meditation is practiced in anthroposophic music therapy, namely sound meditation. It is in equal measure both a source of inspiration and our "daily bread". We listen into a tone, an interval, a sequence of tones, or a scale and try to perceive the intrinsic nature of this tone, interval, sequence or scale. Only when the interval is revealed in this way can it be used as an effective "medicine" in music therapy. Quietude is the prerequisite for such listening, inner and outer quiet. Quietude is required for every kind of meditation and inner contemplation.

Meditative work for the sculptor

Elke Dominik

Alongside daily artistic-meditative work on Rudolf Steiner's sculptural and architectural forms, the meditations "Growing and Withering"[141] and "Seed"[142] can be a helpful accompanying practice for sculptors. Insight into living phenomena is strengthened by concentrating on purely inner processes. Organs are formed for perceiving the reality of the forces of growth and development. A basic requirement for creative sculptural work that draws on the impulses given by Rudolf Steiner is to work together with the life forces.

Meditation on "Growing and Withering":

"The start must be made by turning the attention of our soul towards certain processes in the world surrounding us. Such processes are burgeoning, growing and thriving life on the one hand and all phenomena which are connected with withering, fading and dying away on the other. Such processes are present simultaneously everywhere were human beings turn their eye. And everywhere they also naturally call forth feelings and thoughts in human beings.

But under normal circumstances human beings do not open themselves sufficiently to these feelings and thoughts. They rush much too quickly from one impression to the next for this to be able to happen. It is a matter of turning their attention very deliberately towards these facts. Where they perceive growth and withering of a very specific kind, they must banish everything else from their soul and give themselves over to this impression alone for a brief time.

They will soon be convinced that a feeling which previously flitted through the soul grows in strength so that it takes on a forceful and vigorous form. They must then allow this form of feeling quietly to linger in themselves. They must become very quiet within themselves. They must close themselves off from the rest of the external world and solely follow what their soul says with regard to the fact of growth and withering.

But no one should think that they will get very far by dulling their senses towards the world. First we should look as vividly, as precisely as possible at things. Only then should we give ourselves over to the feelings coming alive in the soul, the thoughts arising. The important thing is to turn our attention to both things in complete inner equilibrium.

If we find the necessary peace and give ourselves over to what comes to life in the soul, we will experience the following after the appropriate time. We will see new kinds of feelings and thoughts arising within us which we did not know beforehand. The more often we turn our attention in this way to something growing, blossoming and flourishing and alternately something which is withering and dying off, the more vivid these feelings will become.

And out of the feelings and thoughts which arise in this way our organs of clairvoyance will develop in the same way that the eyes and ears of the physical body develop through natural forces out of living matter. A very specific form of feeling is associated with growth and development; and another very specific one with withering and dying. But only in the event that the cultivation of these feelings is striven for in the way described.

It is possible to give a reasonably accurate description of what these feelings are like. But everyone can obtain a complete idea of them for themselves by going through these inner experiences. Anyone who has frequently directed their attention to the process of becoming, flourishing and blossoming will feel something distantly akin to the feeling on seeing a sunrise. And out of the process of withering and dying off an experience will result which in the same way can be compared with the slow rise of the moon over the horizon. Both these feelings are two forces which, if they are properly cultivated, can lead to the most significant spiritual effects the more vividly they are developed."

The "seed meditation":

"We lay the small seed from a plant in front of us. The important thing is intensively to think the right thoughts about this unremarkable thing and to develop certain feelings through these thoughts. To begin with, we should be clear what we really see with our eyes. We should describe for ourselves the form, colour and all other characteristics of the seed.

Then think the following. Out of this seed will grow a varied plant when it is planted in the earth. Picture this plant in front of your mind's eye. Construct it in your imagination. And then think: what I am now seeing in my imagination, that is what the forces of the earth and light will later on actually draw forth.

If I had an artificially formed object before me which looked exactly like the seed, so that my eyes could not distinguish it from a real one, no power on earth or of the light could draw forth a plant from it. Anyone who makes this thought very clear to themselves, who experiences it inwardly, will also be able to form the following one with the right feeling.

They will tell themselves: in the seed there already lies in a concealed way – as a force of the whole plant – what will later grow out of it. This force does not lie in the artificial imitation. And yet to my eyes both seem the same. The real seed thus contains something invisible which is not in the imitation. We now direct our feelings and thoughts at this invisible element.[143]

Imagine: this invisible element will later be transformed into the visible plant which I will have before me with its shape and colour. Pursue the thought: the invisible will become visible. If I were unable to think, what will become visible later on could not herald itself to me at this time already.

Let me emphasise emphatically: what we think in this situation also has to be intensively felt. We must in all calmness experience the single thought indicated above without any other thoughts and feelings attaching to it. And we have to give ourselves time so that the thought and the feeling associated with it drill into the soul as it were.

If we can manage to do this in the right way, then after a time we will feel a force in us – perhaps only after many attempts.

And this force will create a new visual perception. The seed will appear as if enclosed in a small cloud of light. It will be experienced in a sensory spiritual way as a kind of flame. Towards the centre of this flame we experience the same kind of feeling as we have when we feel the impression the colour purple makes; towards the edge, the same kind of feeling as we experience with a bluish colour.

In this way there comes to experience what we did not previously see and what has been created by the power of the thought and the feelings we awoke in ourselves. What was not visible to the senses, the plant which will only become visible later on, that is revealed in a spiritually visible way."

Anthroposophic Body Therapy

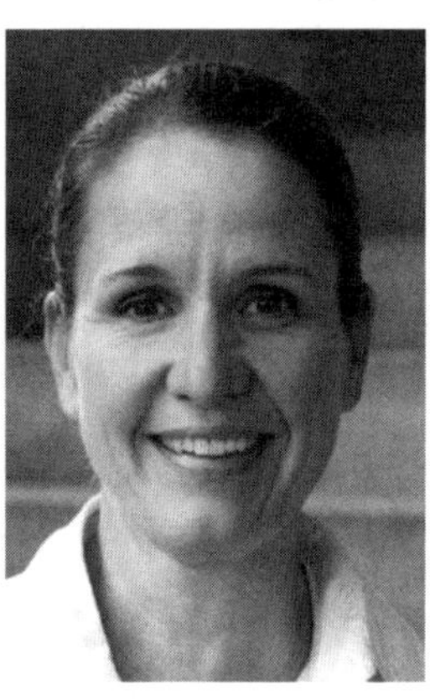

Elma Th. Pressel, non-medical practitioner, body therapist
International Coordination of Anthroposophic Body Therapy
elma.pressel@t-online.de
www.iaabt-medsektion.net

What is the contribution of anthroposophic body therapy in the system of Anthroposophic Medicine?

Anthroposophic body therapy comprises many different therapeutic methods which are initiated by means of movement or touch directly on the human body.

Their common foundation is provided by the extension of medical and therapeutic concepts on the basis of the anthroposophical understanding of the human being as well as the development of therapeutic impulses going back to Rudolf Steiner and Dr med. Ita Wegman.

Their field of activity comprises all parts of society and age groups and can be found in all fields of medicine, outpatient and inpatient, acute care medicine as much as the care of chronically ill patients, rehabilitation to the same extent as independent practice.

In the context of salutogenesis, the methods of anthroposophic body therapy additionally make a significant contribution in the form of health education, stress management and prevention.

What methods are there? How many anthroposophical body therapists are working worldwide?

The following methods are in association with one another at the time of publication of this new edition of the book:

- Hydrotherapy and external treatments: oil dispersion baths as developed by W. Junge and other types (rhythmical baths as developed by Dr med. Ita Wegman, Schnabel bath, surf bath as developed by Liske-Usbeck), wraps and external applications.
- Massages: rhythmical massage therapy as developed by Dr med. Ita Wegman and massage as developed by Dr med. Simeon Pressel.
- Movement therapies: Bothmer gymnastics, Loheland gymnastics and Spacial Dynamics®.

More will be added.

In addition there is a not inconsiderable number of therapists who place their work in a close relationship with the anthroposophic medical movement without working with one of the above methods. There are several working and initiative groups.

There were almost 800 qualified therapists working in rhythmical massage therapy and physiotherapy in 2012, 600 of them in Europe.

For the other methods a precise overall number is difficult

to ascertain since the many different training situations mean that until now it has not been possible to apply comparable criteria.

There is a network to maintain association among therapists, many of whom work alone across the world and feel a connection with the Medical Section.

How is the association of methods in anthroposophic body therapy organised? How is it financed?

The individual methods are organised in independent professional associations.

The impulse to provide a common umbrella for the various methods of body therapy led to the foundation of the "International Association for Anthroposophic Body Therapy" (IAABT) in 2011.

It supports the training and advanced training of medical body therapists who want to extend their work with the methods of anthroposophical spiritual science.

The IAABT campaigns for free choice of therapy and pluralism in medicine, and nationally and internationally supports the legal safeguarding of the various methods of body therapy.

Representatives of the individual methods have the opportunity here to enter into contact with other methods, make an active contribution, and communicate the interests of their own professional group.

Finance

The financing concept is based on the insight and will of the individual person and the associations. It calls for each therapist internationally to provide the national monetary value of one hour of therapy as an annual solidarity contribution for the IAABT and the Coordination in the Medical Section. This is intended to form a foundation for the professional field and its coordination so that they can in future finance themselves independently of the Medical Section.

How are the modes of work and responsibility structures described in this book practised in anthroposophic body therapy?

The mode of work in body therapy is based on the initiative of the individual methods and their representatives. These representatives have a particular spiritual responsibility as set out in this book and are links in community building. This is backed by the Coordination/IKAM and instrumentally supported by the IAABT.

"The healthy social life is found when in the mirror of each human soul the whole community finds its reflection; and when in the community the virtue of each one is living."[144]

How is the next generation supported in anthroposophic body therapy? Where is there training and advanced training?

International specialist conferences on anthroposophic body therapy (formerly "International Conference for Physiotherapy") take place at the Goetheanum in a biennial rhythm. They are a key part of specialist collaboration and exchange between all those working in body therapy in the various specialist areas worldwide. They offer a good opportunity for new entrants to find their bearings. There are various training and advanced training centres for the individual methods. The International Forum for Rhythmical Massage Therapy Training (IFRMTT) meets each year before the annual conference of the Medical Section to work on the basics of the method.

At university level there is the opportunity in Austria, through the collaboration between the Ita Wegman Academy Graz (rhythmical massage therapy) and the Seggau/Graz Interuniversity College for Medical and Therapeutic Specialists, to take a Masters course in complementary, psychosocial and integrative health sciences on an anthroposophical basis.

At Cusanus University in Bernkastel-Kues in Germany, a part-time Bachelors course in the department of therapy sciences started for the first time in the autumn 2014 with rhythmical massage therapy and oil dispersion baths; other body therapy methods will follow later.

How is spiritual substance cultivated in anthroposophic body therapy?

Ecce homo

Feeling weaves
In the heart,

Thinking illuminates
The head,

Will powers
The limbs.

Weaving illumination,
Powerful weaving,
Illuminating power:
That is – the human being.

Rudolf Steiner[145]

The diversity of the activities of this professional group is reflected in the diverse way the individual therapists engage with the different meditations. The warmth meditation[146] links us with all the medical professional groups and the meditation "See in thy Soul power of radiance ..."[147] with the eurythmy therapists and art therapists. The Foundation Stone verse is a sustaining element.

The following meditation "What I speak from my physical body is semblance ..." was given by Rudolf Steiner to Ita Wegman in October 1923 after the conference in Penmaenmawr, Wales:

What I speak from my physical body is semblance –
I must speak from my etheric body,
to penetrate into true reality:

1. You spirits below the earth press on the soles of my feet.
   I stride above you.

2. You spirits of moisture caress my skin
   I press you to all sides.
3. You spirits of the air fill my inner being.
   I unite myself with you.
4. You spirits of warmth ensoul my inner being.
   I live in you.
5. You spirits of the light enspirit my inner being.
   I think with you.
6. You spirits of (chemical) forces subdue my forces.
   I wish to overcome you.
7. You spirits of life deaden my life.
   I await you in death.

Saying this, I am in the etheric body.
And you may come: Colours, tones, words of the etheric world.[148]

Although intended primarily for eurythmists, the following verse is experienced and cultivated as an enrichment also in our professional group:

I seek within

The working of creative forces,
The life of creative powers.
Earth's gravity
Is telling me
Through the word of my feet,
Air's power of form
Is telling me
Through the singing of my hands,
Heaven's strength of light
Is telling me
Through the thinking of my head
How the world in human beings
Speaks, sings, contemplates.

Rudolf Steiner[149]

Furthermore, the meditations of the Samaritan course are cultivated (see page 125 f.). The two mantric verses "Well up o blood ..."[150] and "As long as thou dost feel the pain,..."[151] connect us with the nursing professional group and are also an important component of esoteric deepening for some therapists in the way we handle wounds and pain.

The following verse from Rudolf Steiner can be of help in developing a mindful and calmly spirit-connected attitude in undertaking treatment which takes us completely into the development of the will and thus the courage to heal:

I bear calm within myself,
I bear within myself
The forces which strengthen me.
I want to fill myself
With the warmth of these forces,
I want to pervade myself
With the power of my will.
And I want to feel
How calm spreads
Through all my being
When I strengthen myself
To find calm as
The force within me
Through the power of my striving.

Rudolf Steiner[152]

The courage and will to heal are addressed specifically also in the following text which particularly acknowledges the "earthly" approach of body therapy work while at the same time highlighting the connection with the spirit which characterises our activity within Anthroposophic Medicine:

Seek truly practical material life,
But seek it such that it does not insensitise you
to the spirit at work in it.

Seek the spirit,

But seek it not in supersensory ecstasy,
        out of supersensory egoism,
But seek it
As you would use it selflessly in practical life,
        in the material world.

Apply the ancient principle:
"Spirit is never without matter, matter never
        without spirit" such that you say:
We want to do everything in the light of the spirit,
And we want to seek the light of the spirit such
That it develops warmth for us in our practical work.

Spirit guided by us into matter,
Matter which we work on to
        its revelation,
Through which it shows the spirit within it;
Matter which receives revelation of the spirit through us,
Spirit which is driven towards matter
        through us,
They form the living existence
Which can bring humanity to achieve
        real progress,
To such progress which can only be longed for
        by the best in the profoundest depths
        of souls in our present time.

Rudolf Steiner[153]

Anthropsophic midwives

Christiane Hinderlich

There has been an association of anthroposophic midwives since 2014 which is represented with a coordinator in IKAM. The association works for anthroposophically extended midwifery to support holistic care in an anthroposophical sense through pregnancy, birth and until the end of the first year. To this end this group has as its aim:

- organising conferences for the professional exchange of views among midwives about specialist medical and spiritual subjects and about anthroposophical perspectives on the work of midwives,
- creating spaces to meet for the professional exchange of views and advanced training between midwives and e.g. gynaecologists, paediatricians and nurses,
- supporting and organising conferences on the content of anthroposophically extended midwifery,
- building an up-to-date further training provision for anthroposophically extended midwifery,
- developing certification for midwives in the field of anthroposophically extended midwifery as a quality assurance measure,
- progressing anthroposophically extended care concepts and therapy forms in midwifery,
- developing holistic care concepts in midwifery with the inclusion of anthroposophic medicines,
- supporting scientific research for the evaluation and scientific deepening of subjects related to anthroposophically extended midwifery,
- undertaking public relations work to spread knowledge about anthroposophically extended midwifery.

International Coordination of Anthroposophic Non-medical Practitioners

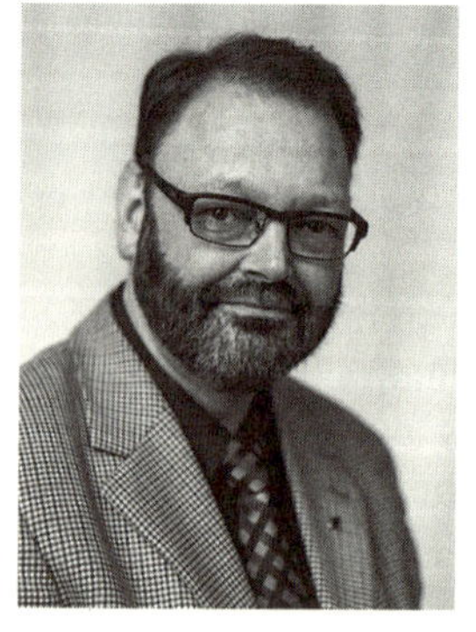

Alexander Schadow, non-medical practitioner in psychotherapy
International Coordination of Anthroposophic Non-medical Practitioners
Professional Association for Anthroposophic Non-medical Practitioners (AGAHP)
verband@agahp.de
www.agahp.de

"We are anthroposophists and we are non-medical practitioners" was the motto of the non-medical practitioners associated with Mr and Mrs Knur who gathered at the Wala premises in 1978 to form an informal working group. In 1992, AGAHP e.V. was founded as the professional association for non-medical practitioners together with the head of the Medical Section, Dr med. Michaela Glöckler. The anthroposophic non-medical practitioners have been represented as a professional group in the Medical Section since that time.

Collaboration with the authorities

In 2008 the German Health Ministry recognised the AGAHP as the representative of anthroposophic non-medical practitioners. With this came the right to propose members for Medicinal Commission C of the Federal Institute for Drugs and Medical Devices BfArM: Markus Pütter and Elisabeth Oelmaier represent the anthroposophic non-medical practitioners on Medicinal Commission C. In 2011, an occupational profile in English of the anthroposophic non-medical practitioner was submitted for the EU-initiated Cambrella project through membership of the European advocacy group for naturopathy/ANME; this professional group is thereby now also present at a European level.

Anthroposophic non-medical practice

The first IKAM professional group coordinator for anthroposophic non-medical practice was Renate Künne. She was succeeded in 2014 by her deputy as professional group coordinator until then, Alexander Schadow.

The term "anthroposophic non-medical practice" as designation for the activity of anthroposophic non-medical practitioners goes back to an agreement between Werner Schmötzer as the first executive director of AGAHP, the representatives of the Society of Anthroposophic Physicians in Germany / GAÄD and the Medical Section. At the same time it was agreed that the occupational designation "Anthroposophic Medicine" would be reserved for physicians.

The international professional group for anthroposophic non-medical practice also includes groupings of persons working in non-medical practice who want to work anthroposophically and are seeking contact with the Goetheanum.

Qualification and certification

The qualification in anthroposophic non-medical practice is undertaken through the AGAHP-accredited lecturers in anthroposophic non-medical practice (AGAHP)®, particularly in the subjects: professional studies in and professional esotericism of anthroposophic non-medical practice. The maintenance, further development and communication of these core competences is the particular task of the association's school ANTHROPOS-SOPHIA. Anthroposophic non-medical practice as the activity of anthroposophic non-medical practitioners can be certified by AGAHP.

The AGAHP handbook, the guiding principles and the occupational profile of the anthroposophic non-medical practitioner as well as the statutes of the AGAHP can be found on our website: www.agahp.de.

Meditative life

The path to the profession of non-medical practitioner is a very individual one marked by the particular features of a person's biography. We see the karmic encounter between patient and non-medical practitioner based on personal initiative as a key element in the healing process.

Cultivation of the anthroposophical path of schooling combined with insight into the karmic origin of our own will to heal is thus also a central concern for non-medical practitioners and an important part of the training. Traditionally the weekly verse is read at the start of every meeting of anthroposophic non-medical practitioners, often also – to develop an earth-encompassing awareness – together with the corresponding verse for the southern hemisphere.

At each conference of the professional group and the non-medical practitioners' association Arbeitsgemeinschaft Anthroposophischer Heilpraktiker / AGAHP there is also always a meeting of Class members in which the specific esotericism of the professional group is cultivated.

There is no general mantra for non-medical practitioners. But I would like to draw attention to two mantras which are of great importance in non-medical practitioner circles and are meditated by many colleagues. The first one is the mantra given in the Pastoral Medicine Course: "I will go the path ..."

I will go the path,
Which dissolves the elements into process
And leads me downwards to the Father
Who sends the illness as balance to karma.
And leads me upwards to the spirit
Who guides the soul in error to attainment of freedom.
Christ leads downwards and upwards
Harmoniously creating spirit human being in earthly human being.

Rudolf Steiner[154]

Since the profession of the non-medical practitioner has always also included a spiritual and pastoral component, many colleagues feel an affinity with it.

The other one is the warmth meditation (see page 111 f.) which is cultivated by many non-medical practitioners. In this context it is important for us to feel connected with all the other anthroposophical professional groups out of our own ego-consciousness in this way.

Coordination of Nutrition

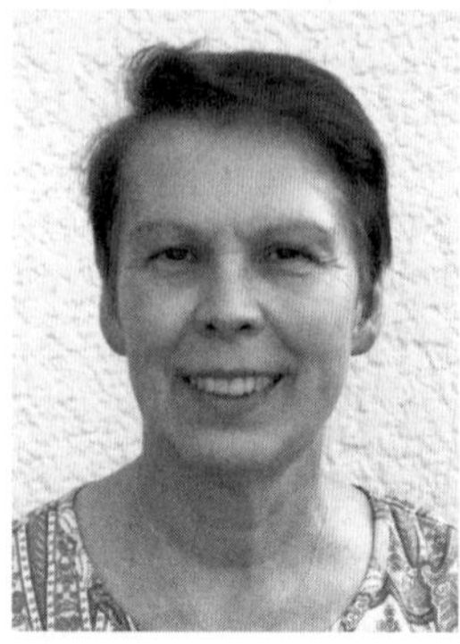

Dr sc. agr. Petra Kühne
Coordination of Nutrition
www.ak-ernaehrung.de

What is the contribution of anthroposophic nutritional research in the system of Anthroposophic Medicine?

Nutrition is an important element of prevention as well as therapy (diets). Here the importance of nutrition has only recently been recognised again. If up to the middle of the twentieth century there were many diets and nutritional therapies, new findings about their minimal impact ("light diet") as well as medicinal treatment sidelined those existing diets. In the last decades there has been a growing recognition of the preventive importance of nutrition (e.g. choice of fats for cardiovascular health, cancer-preventing foods, importance of dietary fibre). Similarly there was the development of new nutritional recommendations e.g. for type 2 diabetes, rheumatism and so on.

Anthroposophic nutrition is based on recommendations for biodynamic quality in farming, the anthroposophical understanding of the world and nature and thus a certain concept of quality. There are not, however, fixed rules but this is individualised nutrition which requires the individual to take responsibility. The anthroposophic nutritional movement consists of nutritional consultants, chefs in various institutions and a few nutritional researchers.

Is the association organised? How is it financed?

An association currently only exists in the form of individual groups mainly in Germany, Switzerland and the Netherlands as well as a section group in the School of Spiritual Science at the Goetheanum jointly between the Medical and Agricultural sections, as well as the Nutritional Research Working Group in Bad Vilbel. There is no common finance yet, the participating people cover their own costs.

How is the next generation supported? What training, further training and advanced training provisions are there?

The Nutritional Research Working Group (AKE) has offered part-time further training in anthroposophic nutrition since 2007 in Frankfurt am Main. In the Netherlands there are courses for anthroposophic nutritional consultants, in Switzerland for people working in group catering.

International Coordination of Medical Training

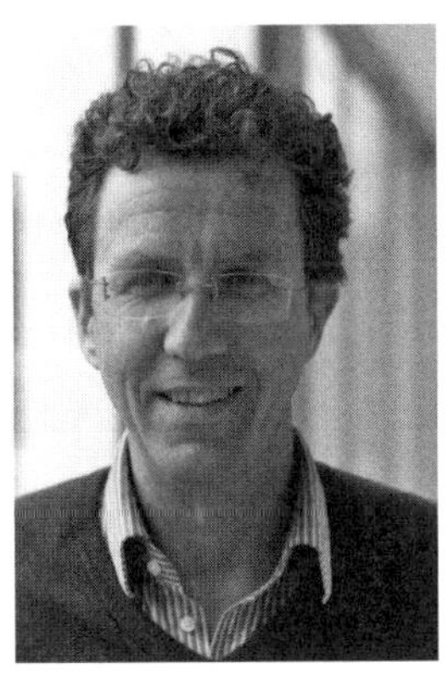

Dr med. Jan Feldmann
International Coordination of Anthroposophic Medical Training
janfeldmann@yahoo.de
info@akademie-havelhoehe.de

Organisational form of the professional field

There is meanwhile anthroposophic medical training courses in over 20 countries worldwide. The overwhelming majority are the result of national initiatives in their respective countries, most of them as training courses lasting several years; their successful conclusion leads to approval as an anthroposophic physician.

Once a year there is a meeting of lecturers and training directors from many countries during the international conference at the Goetheanum. The aim of this trainer conference is to develop and promote the quality and professionalisation of trainers and training courses. Conferences themes are methodology, didactics and content of anthroposophic teaching in medicine.

Teaching in Anthroposophic Medicine is being professionalised through group work, lectures, patient demonstrations, interactive teaching and learning, case discussion with colleagues, accreditation processes and evaluation. Trainers and those physicians who want to become trainers can participate in this "Teaching the Teacher" programme.

Tasks of the coordinator

Coordination of the professional field, supporting initiatives, community building among physicians working in training, evaluation of training, participation in the International Coordination of Anthroposophic Medicine (IKAM).

Long-term goals

Training, further training and advanced training

- Establishment of advanced training provision in all countries with anthroposophic medical training.
- Development of further standards of education.
- Collaboration and networking with other anthroposophic medical approaches.

Quality

- Accreditation of training initiatives in all countries with an anthroposophic medical training.
- Further development of competence profiles (certification).

Projects

- Drawing up literature on the methodology and didactics of teaching in Anthroposophic Medicine.
- Development of an accreditation procedure.

International Coordination of Anthroposophic Specialist Physicians

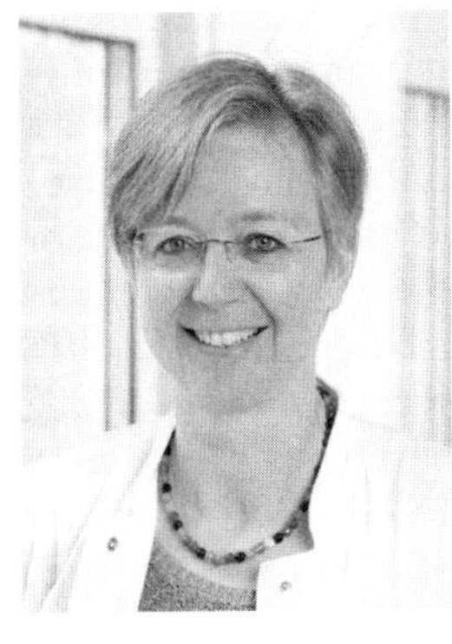

Dr med. Marion Debus
International Coordination of Anthroposophic Specialist Physicians
marion.debus@havelhoehe.de
www.havelhoehe.de

The "Specialist Physicians" coordination field serves to strengthen and support the specialist impulses in our medical movement. The whole of the anthroposophic clinic impulse and many other aspects, the future of AM in an environment of increasing specialisation and sub-specialisation are associated with this.

Specialist groups

Specialist working groups are currently mostly represented in Germany with individual participants from other European countries. There are working groups for neurology, paediatrics, school physicians, dermatology, cardiology, gynaecology, pulmonology, orthopaedics, ENT, dental medicine as well as a "medical pharmaceutical working group to obtain an understanding of medicines in psychiatric illness". Therapists and pharmacists as well as interested general practitioners and medical students are firmly integrated in some groups while others prefer that specialists only take part.

Many groups, which meet twice a year as a rule, are very active in the development of treatment concepts, book and journal publications, organisation of advanced specialist training in the context of the GAÄD and the Medical Section, or of conferences on specific subjects, e.g. the annual conference of the Medical Section by the cardiologists in 2013 and the Easter conference of the GAÄD in 2015 by the neurologists.

The groups are individually grown structures which, although they are largely open to new participants, are not currently generally transparent with regard to contact persons, ways of working, conditions of participation as well as time and place of meetings. The individual working groups have been asked for this information and it will be published shortly on the websites of the GAÄD and Medical Section – on the latter also in English translation – as well as in *Merkurstab*. Access to the working groups for interested persons – also internationally – is thus to be made easier. The Specialist section in *Merkurstab* will offer a forum to report in brief about the most important issues or work results in the respective specialist groups.

Support for new specialist groups

Working groups have not yet formed in some very important specialisms, e.g. anaesthetics, surgery, urology, radiology/radiotherapy. Other groups, for example ophthalmology, have dissolved for various reasons, sometimes after many years of work. In the case of the paediatrics, gynaecology and oncology specialist groups, the work was largely focused on the preparation of corresponding GAÄD further training and only any longer takes place in this context. Here correspondingly interested physicians are to be brought together in the future and inactive working groups to be given new impulses.

As a first step, the orthopaedics specialist group was refounded in October 2014 after a gap of several years and will now meet twice a year at the Havelhöhe community hospital. A palliative medicine working group will also meet for the first time in the near future.

Support for young talent

As part of the Academy Day of the GAÄD in Kassel on 14 May 2015 on the subject "Improving advanced training in anthroposophic clinics and practices", there will also be a working group on the subject of specialist training in order to enter into dialogue with young assistants about their questions and wishes with regard to possible specialist training.

Support for the content of the Anthromedics project through the specialist working groups

Specialism-related and disease-specific introductory texts as part of the planned online textbook part will be written by representatives of the relevant specialist groups and thus contribute to the internationalisation of the impulse as a result of the work in the specialist groups.

Anthroposophic dentists

Rudolf Völker

The Working Group of Anthroposophic Dentists was founded in 1957 by a small group of enthusiastic and energetic colleagues associated with Hermann Lauffer, Wolfram Kern and Erich Liehr who largely carried this impulse to the turn of the millennium. Alongside the work on the basics and the tutorial work in regional working groups during this period, various joint activities were undertaken with monthly or quarterly meetings such as the rather more informal conferences at Kloster Bernstein, the annual conferences at the Filder Clinic, specialist conferences at WALA and WELEDA, and St John's Tide conferences in various locations.

Other activities of the Working Group, which alongside the original group in Stuttgart had various regional offshoots in Oldenburg, Holland and Leipzig, included collaboration with eurythmy therapists (among other things, Hermann Lauffer for example worked for many years as a lecturer in eurythmy therapy training in Stuttgart and Hamburg), nutritionists (Dr Renzenbrink, Dr Kühne), speech therapists (Dr Padovan) and physicians (integration of the Working Group as a specialist group in the Society of Anthroposophic Physicians in Germany/GAÄD). Long before German reunification there were contacts for more than 30 years between the Stuttgart group and colleagues in the then GDR with annual meetings and instrumental material and specialist support.

During the early period of the then reformist Witten University, our colleagues Lauffer, Liehr, Runte and Schwerdtfeger in collaboration with Prof. Rotgans held introductory courses in anthroposophic dentistry and with the students visited the Filder Clinic and the companies Wala and Weleda. A medicine list, the "Dental Compendium" which has undergone constant revision to the present day, was prepared in five years of continuous work in weekend meetings and annual one-week closed conferences. Michael Striebel presented the first finished copy at a conference in Dornach in 1985. Our colleague Thomas Höhnle subsequently continued with the work.

From 1985 onwards, an international dental conference was then held in Dornach at two-yearly intervals. This impulse was subsequently replaced in 2007 under the overall direction of Wolfgang Güldenstern by the joint preparation of a curriculum for training dentists and dental students in Anthroposophic Medicine. This was held from 2010 to 2013 in six parts in Kassel, Filderstadt, Berlin-Havelhöhe and Dornach with more than 60 participants from seven countries and on 12 May 2012 it successfully laid a foundation stone for the continued existence of this community with the certificate "Internal Approval in Anthroposophic Dentistry" for twelve new graduates.

This impulse is being carried on so that continuous further training can be assured; new colleagues can be reached through a new edition of the curriculum; international collaboration, e.g. with the French, Dutch, Italian and South American colleagues can be intensified; and the collaboration with our medical colleagues can also be extended.

Motto of the Working Group of Anthroposophic Dentists

Dental enamel is the substance which the organism forms in its earthly development which has grown most physical. The cells which form it, the adamantoblasts, die off after they have completed their task and make their forces available for thinking activity. To this extent work on the dental organ occupies a special place within medicine since we dentists are mostly forced to use alloplastic materials when a tooth is damaged: if preventive possibilities (taking responsibility ourselves for diet and dental care, developing the appropriate awareness at all ages, conservative and preventive teeth brushing and medication) were not adequately recognised and successfully implemented, real recovery (*restitutio ad integrum*) in the treatment of dental substances can no longer be achieved.

Especially against this background – and the discomfort which it often causes in patients who see themselves confronted with the irreversibility of physical pathways – the unity of our work, which superficially takes place essentially at a physical level, with the spiritual aspect is always a concern for us dentists. Our meetings therefore start and end with words from Rudolf Steiner's "Truth Wrought Words" which represent an intense meditation on the close and indivisible connection between matter and spirit in every situation of life and reflect the call on us to act against the ever-present spiritual background:

Seek truly practical material life,
But seek it such that it does not insensitise you
 to the spirit at work in it.
Seek the spirit,
But seek it not in supersensory ecstasy,
 out of supersensory egoism,
But seek it
As you would use it selflessly in practical life,
 in the material world.

Apply the ancient principle:
"Spirit is never without matter, matter never
 without spirit" such that you say:

We want to do everything in the light of the spirit,
And we want to seek the light of the spirit such
That it develops warmth for us in our practical work.

Spirit guided by us into matter,
Matter which we work on to its revelation,
Through which it shows the spirit within it;
Matter which receives revelation of the spirit through us,
Spirit which is driven towards matter through us,
They form the living existence
Which can bring humanity to achieve real progress,
To such progress which can only be longed for
by the best in the profoundest depths
of souls in our present time.

Rudolf Steiner[155]

Working Group of National Associations for and General Representative Bodies of Anthroposophic Medicine – Group of National Coordinators for Anthroposophic Medicine / GNCAM

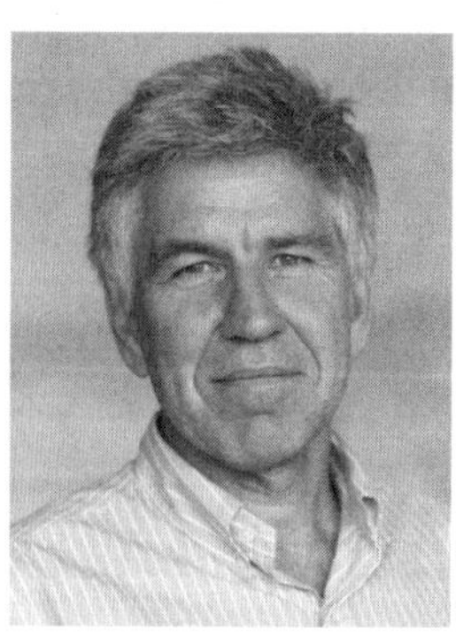

Dr med. Stefan Geider
Representative of GNCAM,
Medical Section Coordinator UK
s.geider@camphillwellbeing.org.uk
www.cahsc.org

National representative bodies of the anthroposophic medical movement

There are some countries in which there is a general representative body of Anthroposophic Medicine. Because countries reflect on a small scale what must be done worldwide on a supranational level: the perception and further development of the concerns of Anthroposophic Medicine.

Such a representation exists in the following countries:

Chile: Asociación de Medicina Antroposófica de Chile
Germany: Dachverband Anthroposophische Medizin in Deutschland / DAMiD, www.damid.de
New Zealand: New Zealand Association of Anthroposophic Doctors (NZAAD), www.anthroposophy.org.nz
Netherlands: Antroposofischer Verein in den Niederlanden, Medizinische Sektion in den Niederlanden, www.antroposofie.nl/hogeschool/gezondheidszorg/
Sweden: LAOM – Läkarföreningen för Antroposofisk Orienterad Medicin
Hungary: Dr med. Henrik Szöke
United Kingdom: Anthroposophic Medical Association, Dr med. Stefan Geider
USA: Physicians Association for Anthroposophic Medicine, www. paam.net

Form of working

Since 2009, the delegates of these national representative bodies have been meeting during the annual conference of the Medical Section to exchange experiences and discuss common concerns and work goals.

Projects

Providing a translation into English of "Individual Paediatrics" by Georg Soldner and Rudolf Steiner's medical lectures. The former project was a new translation and the latter had as its goal to complete the series and revise previous translations. Other translations are at the planning stage, particularly with regard to the Anthromedics project.

International Coordination of Age Culture and Elderly Care

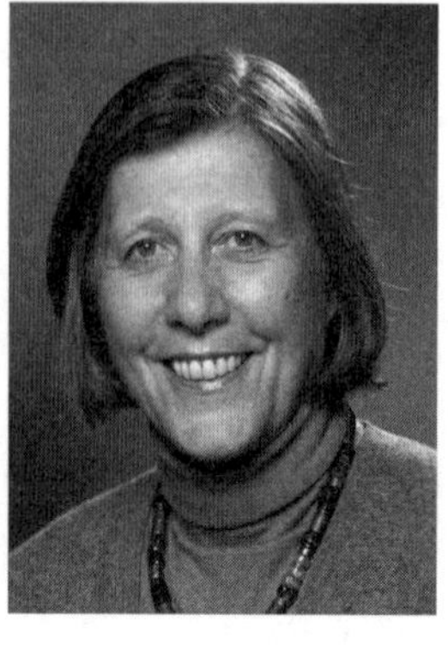

Sabine Ringer
Director of Haus Morgenstern, Stuttgart
International Coordination of Age Culture and Elderly Care
sabine.ringer@haus-morgenstern.de
www.haus-morgenstern.de

A new coordination field introduces itself

The Nikodemus Werk e.V. was founded in 1977 as an organisation with its origins in the movement for religious renewal "The Christian Community" and anthroposophy. The "Werk" currently has 30 member establishments in Germany; their staff have as their goal to implement the spiritual impulse of anthroposophical elderly care in everyday life and to deepen it further (www.nikodemuswerk.de). We see ourselves in the meantime as an international professional association for age culture.

So far there are individual personal connections with other European countries and with Asia.

The Nikodemus Werk also sees itself as a forum for:

- reciprocal consultation and support
- building and extending networks for a forward-looking age culture
- developing contemporary, spiritually extended forms of work, life and learning
- advice on quality questions
- involvement in researching and answering the current questions of humanity, particularly about the meaning of illness, old age, dying and death.

There are two regional groups in Germany, South and North, which support our semi-annual meetings in spring and autumn. There are regular specialist conferences on subjects such as nutrition, building services, care and quality assurance for staff at which the everyday tasks are deepened in their content.

There are meanwhile three specialist schools for anthroposophically oriented elderly care (Frankfurt, Dortmund, Stuttgart – also see below: www.fachseminar-altenpflege.de/links).

Our own quality mark was developed in the course of the legislation for elderly care.

In the general meetings of members we can strengthen our impulse together and exchange views about the sources which we have developed for ourselves. The realisation of the spiritual impulses from anthroposophy and the Christian Community is as manifold as the people who work with them. Each establishment can make its own choices and can decide, for example, whether it wishes to obtain the Nikodemus quality mark. This means that each establishment is truly individual and it is anthroposophy and/or the Christian Community which is the unifying element. The board works as instructed by the general meeting of members, there are "owners" for the individual tasks.

There are currently the following projects:

- Combining the mark of the Nikodemus Werk with Anthro Med® is currently being examined
- Advice and support for establishments in crisis situations
- Representation in "Der Paritätische", in DAMiD (www.damid.de) and in Anthropoi
- Establishment of an entrepreneurial company
- Development of an ownership concept for limited company shares managed in trust
- Establishment of a social fund for the health promotion of staff
- Social policy lobbying to reform the PTV (care assessments)
- Ensuring young talent in specialist and management functions
- Advice for new initiatives

In order to manage these tasks, the directors who until then worked on an honorary basis were given benefits in 2012. At the general meeting of members in 2014, the development of the "Werk" was worked on in the context of the seven rhythms, while current legislative developments were discussed at the autumn meeting.

Basic understanding

In our basic understanding there is a deep meaning to old age as a "new" biographical phase of life: old age not only challenges people to come to terms with the life which lies behind them but also to identify their lasting spiritual qualities – the fruits of their life. It is particularly through the struggles of age that key abilities for the future are developed. It is our aim to support this development through creating a living environment in which the focus is on the individual. In view of waning physical strength and the emotional crises arising as a result, we understand aging as an intensive developmental process which is of value for the elderly person and the whole of society.

The elderly person takes their abilities, newly acquired through the need for care, with them across the threshold of death into the spiritual world. In the anthroposophical understanding of the world and human beings they thereby form the basis for a new life on earth.

What are the most urgent problems on which the Nikodemus Werk is working?

The struggle for a leadership structure which brings the individual nature of an establishment to expression and yet contains the voluntary impulse to find oneself on a spiritual level. But membership numbers have been stagnating for years. In some establishments questions of transition and succession have to be solved, identity questions of the Werk, building trust among one another, professionalisation with chief executives released for that task is being tried out. What keeps us together as NW: We are always striving for a common identity.

Recruiting staff in the field of elderly care is currently and will be in coming years a task which must be tackled if we take demographic developments seriously. The profession of geriatric nurse is unique worldwide and is congruent in its structure with the concerns of the Nikodemus Werk. Involvement in improving the framework conditions (staffing ratio, pay, recognition ...) and communication of the spiritual dimension of this profession can and must be done by anthroposophy.

What structures are used to work on these problems?

The regional groups can allow one another a reciprocal deeper insight and discuss matters with and support one another. Meetings between colleagues are held as part of audits. Personal meetings form the basis for building trust.

We have so far been able to develop an alternative audit procedure which demonstrates individual responsibility and forms of participation instead of questions of control. We see the audit requirements of the authorities also as a consciousness strengthening element for our work.

The Nikodemus Werk wishes to be actively involved in developing an "age culture" through investigating and answering the great questions of humanity in the present time, for example: what is the meaning of illness, dying and death in old age?

Appropriate contemporary social and management structures have to be developed in establishments catering for the elderly so that the opportunity arises "for each person voluntarily to do what lies in their calling in accordance with the measure of their abilities and strength".[156]

From our guiding principles: "The Nikodemus Werk forms a vessel which incorporates spiritual impulses out of which strength can flow to the individual members which they require to cope with everyday life and for their own development." The connection with the Medical Section has been desired for many years; the fundamental questions of an age culture have to be worked on. We would be very pleased about contact with establishments at home and abroad so that this coordination field becomes well anchored within the Section.

European Federation of Patients' Associations for Anthropopsophic Medicine (EFPAM)

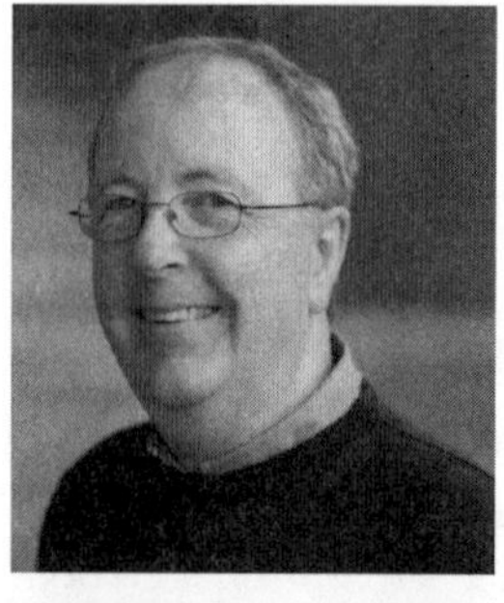

René de Winter
President and coordinator of the European Federation of Patients' Associations for Anthroposophic Medicine
efpam.europe@gmail.com
www.efpam.eu

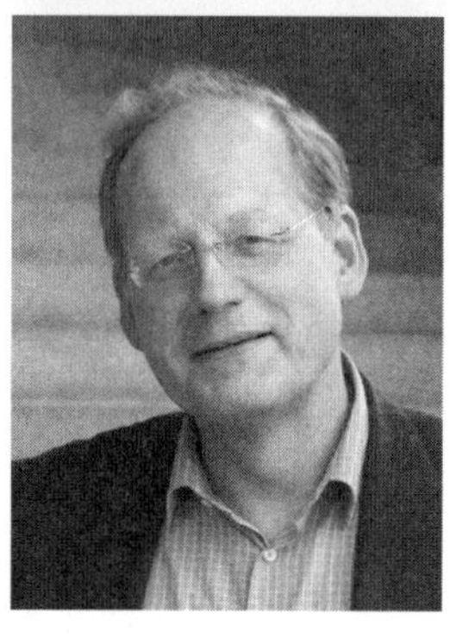

Dr med. Stefan Schmidt-Troschke
gesundheit aktiv
International Coordination of Patient Organisations
www.gesundheit-aktiv.de

For how long has EFPAM been in existence? How many member associations does the patient umbrella association have? How is it organised?

EFPAM was founded on 3 October 2000 in Dornach after many years of preparation. EFPAM currently has 15 full members (national patient associations), of which twelve are in EU countries (Belgium, Denmark, Germany, Finland, France, Italy, Netherlands, Austria, Romania, Sweden, Spain, United Kingdom) and three in non-EU countries (Iceland, Norway, Switzerland).

EFPAM is an association under Alsatian law with its registered office in Strasbourg/FR. Its highest body is the assembly; the board is elected annually by the members.

Members:

- Austria: Verein für ein anthroposophisch erweitertes Heilwesen e.V.
- Belgium: VITA é SANA Vereniging voor Antroposofische Gezondheidszorg vzw / Association pour les Soins de Santé Anthroposophique asbl
- Denmark: Foreningen till støtte for Antroposofisk Læge-Kunst (FALK)
- Finland: Antroposofisen lääketieteen yhdistys ry. (ALY)
- France: Association de Patients de la Médecine anthroposophique (APMA)
- Germany: Gesundheit aktiv, anthroposophische Heilkunst e.V.
- Iceland: Grös og listir – Félag um mannspekilækningar
- Italy: Associazione Italiana dei Pazienti della Medicina Antroposofica (AIPMA)
- Netherlands: Antroposana, patiëntenvereniging voor antroposofische gezondheidszorg
- Norway: Foreningen for Antroposofisk Lege Kunst (FALK)
- Romania: antrosana Romania
- Spain: anthrosana en España – Asociacíon de patientes para un sistema sanitario ampliado antroposóficamente
- Sweden: Föreningen för Antroposofisk Läkekonst (FALK)
- Switzerland: anthrosana, Verein für anthroposophisch erweitertes Heilwesen
- United Kingdom: Patients and Friends of Anthroposophical Medicine (PAFAM)

Associated member

- Canada: Association de Patients de la Médecine anthroposophique au Québec (APMAQ)

What is the mission of EFPAM?

Our missions statement is:

- to support citizens to increase awareness of and responsibility for quality of life and health care through advocating self-

determination, freedom of therapy choice and pluralism in medicine
- by cooperating with other organisations in the field of pluralism in medicine and representing the national associations of patients who use Anthroposophic Medicine in Europe, make their interests known to the authorities
- based on the respect for the dignity of the human being, fundamental human rights and responsibility for nature
- contributing to enable good health for all European citizens.

Aims:

- To represent the views and interests of people who want to use Anthroposophic Medicine in all its forms, besides or instead of other forms of medicine, in particular in the light of the individual right to self-determination.
- To act as interlocutor for European, international and national institutions and to ascertain that policy makers within these institutions are kept well-informed of the wishes and needs of users of Anthroposophic Medicine.
- To promote the development and the cultural and legal recognition of Anthroposophic Medicine in all its forms.
- To promote the recognition and inclusion of the rights of users of Anthroposophic Medicine in all its forms in present and future national and international law.
- To promote and sustain the inclusion of all forms of Anthroposophic Medicine in the various national and private health insurance schemes, on the basis of equality of all citizens.
- To promote patients' awareness of and responsibility for the preservation and promotion of their own health.
- To encourage research into Anthroposophic Medicine with all appropriate means.
- To promote knowledge of Anthroposophic Medicine and contribute towards its preventive and curative applications.

What structures are used to work on these tasks?

- Cooperation with anthroposophical organisations and establishments in the health sector as well as with CAM organisations, forming of alliances, networking, observing European health policy, particularly with regard to its applicability for the registration of anthroposophic medical products (AMPs) and the availability of AMPs within the EU.

- Cooperation with the Anthroposophic Medical Products – European Policy Working Group (AMP-EPWG) to retain AMPs.
- Cooperation in EUROCAM: pursuit of the statutory recognition of Anthroposophic Medicine and its medicines in Europe, together with other methods of complementary medicine.

Coordination of Public Relations

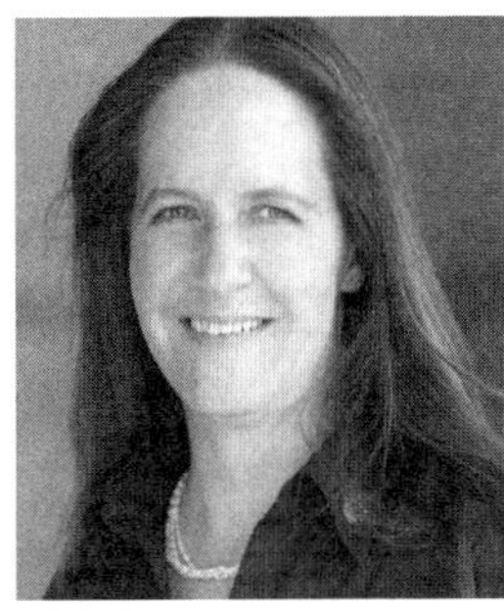

Heike Sommer MA
Coordination of Public Relations
heike.sommer@medsektion-goetheanum.ch
www.medsektion-goetheanum.org

Maintaining association and learning from one another

The anthroposophic medical movement has for many years been developing into an internationally cooperating network whose members are at work in more than 64 countries. Public relations work therefore requires an international and regional form. Then there is the additional factor at a political level that within the countries, but also in Europe, campaigning for pluralism of methods, free choice of therapy and patience competence still requires a great deal of support.

Pooling and distributing information

Here the common focus is on intercommunication and information between specialists, but also to enhance the extent to which Anthroposophic Medicine is known among the public as an integrative therapy system, to raise its profile. After all, Anthroposophic Medicine can look back on a European tradition which has grown organically over decades with proven therapies and medicines. On a practical level this means that public relations work must, on the one hand, ensure the availability of the working documents and, on the other, engage in networking. This is done via the following channels:

- Website: the five-language website is constantly being developed to make the information available to everyone who wants to have it.
- Social media: in order to address the younger generation, the basic information is available on all common social networks such as Facebook, Twitter and Google+ where there is also the opportunity for dialogue and exchange.
- Mailings, newsletters: for rapid international communication and targeted information about current events, special happenings and relevant AM policy content.
- Ebooks: print is engaged in a process of change to which we want to retain the connection. Furthermore, we have found that there is a clear need and want to keep our most important books and new publications quickly available for our international working community and community of members in this way at a reasonable cost.

Further goals

The coordination centre further offers PR consultation, the preparation of PR and multimedia concepts, the coordination of AM information materials and the further development of our international online presence also in the form of new websites or others which through a relaunch have adapted to new technical possibilities. The future viability and sustainability of this coordinating activity lies in the increased visibility of the movement as a whole and its services among the public, being able rapidly and in good time to respond to the current social conditions and react to their requirements.

Joint work on a "breviary"

Michaela Glöckler

The breviary as a constant companion on the inner path is an integral part of the priesthood. For physicians, Steiner in the course for young physicians recommends meditative work "where possible and as needed". Thus the question about an authoritative breviary is just as reasonable as the question about individual meditations to strengthen attentiveness and empathy on the therapeutic path. It is also worthwhile asking whether the structure and order of the medical meditations do not also contain profound references to the seasons in which they were given by Steiner to the physicians, nurses and special needs teachers: starting with the warmth meditation in the autumn of 1923 (see page 111 f.), of which we know for certain that it was worked on at this time by the medical students and young physicians to whom it had been given, the medical path goes via the Raphael imagination[157] for the lectures in preparation of the Christmas Conference at the Goetheanum through to the mystery compositions[158] which also include the publication of the medical mysteries and in the context of which Ita Wegman asked Steiner for a special meditation for nursing. There followed the Christmas Conference with the refounding of the School of Spiritual Science as a mystery school and the Medical Section which was looked after by Rudolf Steiner und Ita Wegman. In the Foundation Stone Meditation for the General Anthroposophical Society, the focus is on the healing task of anthroposophy for the cultural life of people in general. The meditation ends in the commemoration of the Christmas happening at the turning point of time (see page 158 ff.).

In parallel to the Easter course for young physicians, Rudolf Steiner gave lectures for the members of the Anthroposophical

Society on Rosicrucianism and the modern principle of initiation, as well as the lectures: "Easter as a Chapter in the Mystery Wisdom of Humanity".[159] Both lecture cycles, held in parallel, deal with crucial parts of a spiritual medicine and show how closely connected the medical path is with the general anthroposophical one with regard to their therapeutic mission. Between Whitsun and St John's Tide, the Agricultural Course[160] for healing the earth was then held in Koberwitz and directly after St John's Tide the Curative Education Course for physicians and special needs teachers in Dornach, followed by the Pastoral Medicine Course in September 1924.[161] That concluded the "medical year". All these lectures contain indispensable material for suggestions and guidance regarding the spiritual development of the specific professions. Working up this material remains a task to be done.

In parallel to writing down the Michael Letters and the Persephone Mystery, the manuscript for the book *Extending Practical Medicine* is completed with Ita Wegman. That also lays out the "system of Anthroposophic Medicine", the continued development of which will be the task of many generations of physicians to come.

In what follows, the central meditations for physicians will be put in the context of the medical and therapeutic work as a whole in a kind of "weekly breviary". An arrangement was selected in this respect which has been repeatedly taken up by individual co-workers since the annual conferences at the Goetheanum from 1998 to 2004, throughout which aspects of meditative schooling were also a constant theme.

It offers the opportunity to bring to mind with clear regularity and in a weekly rhythm the central work impulses of the anthroposophic medical movement and the professional groups active in it. Here the qualities of the individual weekdays are also helpful in keeping this work filled with life.

Sunday / sun

The meditative path indicated by Rudolf Steiner in the medical field starts with the so-called warmth meditation.

Steiner gave it to a group of students – the "young physicians" – who had asked him about qualities of "morality and love" in medicine (cf. page 111 f.). It starts with the question: How do I find the good? The question about giving and receiving good treatment, about the good physician and the good physician-patient relationship lies at the heart of every "good" medical system. Through the warmth meditation the physician learns to know their own etheric body in a differentiated way, and to strengthen their moral qualities. This meditation also supports interdisciplinary collaboration and conveys the warmth which the anthroposophic medical movement needs to live. In pursuing this initial question, the meditation leads to awareness of the four sources of etheric forces:

The warmth ether works strongly in the interpersonal realm, in humanity's warmth centre, in the Christ being who mediates and permeates everything. The light ether radiates from the heart, the tone ether from the lower body/metabolic realm, while the life ether stirs in the head's life and thinking activity. Moral ideals are what warm and illuminate us, inspire and enliven our work. New etheric forces are needed for healing and culturally creative deeds.

For decades this meditation has found a home wherever Anthroposophic Medicine and special needs education have been taken up and practiced out of a spiritual impulse. Today it can thus be seen and experienced as the spiritual soil in which research and practice of Anthroposophic Medicine can take root. Anyone who wish to take up this meditation for themselves may best have it explained to them by an anthroposophic physician who works with it and – as with other meditative material – write it out personally for themselves.

Just as the sun is the core of warmth and light, but also the source of all life on earth, so the warmth meditation mediates the path to experiencing the soul and spirit sun in a way that gives orientation for therapeutic work.

The warmth meditation

Preparation: How do I find the good?

1. Can I think the good?

   I cannot think the good.
   Thinking is brought about by my etheric body.
   My etheric body works in the fluid of my body.
   Therefore I do not find the good in the fluid of the body.

2. Can I feel the good?

   I can indeed feel the good; however it is not made present by me if I only feel it.
   Feeling is brought about by my astral body.
   My astral body works in the aeriform of my body.
   Therefore in the aeriform of my body I cannot find the good that exists through me.

3. Can I will the good?

   I can will the good.
   Willing is brought about by my ego.
   My ego works in the warmth ether of my body.
   Therefore in the warmth I can physically realise the good.

I feel my humanity in my warmth

1. I feel light in my warmth.

   (Take care that this sensation of light emerges in the region where the physical heart lies)

2. I feel, sounding, world substance in my warmth.

   (Take care that the specific sensation of tone goes from the lower body towards the head but spreading out into the whole body)

3. I feel in my head cosmic life stirring in my warmth.

(Take care that the specific sensation of life spreads from the head to the whole body)

Rudolf Steiner[162]

Monday / moon

The moon stands in a specially coordinated relationship with the earth and the sun, giving rise, for example, to sun and moon eclipses. Moon forces imbue all regenerative processes and natural fertility with rhythm. Human beings too retain during life the 25-hour rhythm of the moon's daily orbit of the earth as an underlying factor of our circadian biorhythm, acquiring the latter only during childhood from the sun as the external time-giver. The first meditation from the Christmas course for young physicians leads us into an experience of the healing spirituality of nature. This meditation connects, in particular, physicians and pharmacists in inner work.

Ye healing spirits
You unite
With sulphur's blessing
In the ethereal fragrance;

You come to life
In Mercury's upward striving,
Dewdrop
Of growing
And becoming.

You come to rest
In the earth salt
Which nourishes the root
In the soil.

I will unite
The knowledge of my soul

With fire of the flower's fragrance;

I will bestir
The life of my soul
On the glistening drop of leafy morning;

I will make strong
The being of my soul with the all hardening salt
With which the earth
With loving care nurtures the root.

Rudolf Steiner[163]

Tuesday / Mars

The two-year rhythm of the Mars orbit has the special quality of a great, macrocosmic breath in which Mars at one point wanders far out into the realm beyond the sun between the asteroids and Jupiter, then subsequently approaches the earth so closely that it enters the planetary sphere between Venus and Mercury in the realm between the sun and the earth. This dynamic corresponds to the battle, mediated by the rhythmical system, between light and heaviness, as Rudolf Steiner sets out in the last meditation in the Christmas course for young physicians. Here we see the daily battle between health and illness, between matter with its "might of heaviness" and spirit with its "power of radiance".

In this meditation we are led to an understanding of the medicinal value of each substance or of an internal process within us. Rudolf Steiner brings this exercise into especially close connection with eurythmy therapy. It also inspires the other art therapies which work in a healing way within this interplay of forces.

See in thy soul
    Power of radiance
Feel in thy body
    Might of heaviness
In the power of radiance
    Shines spirit-I

In the might of heaviness
    God's spirit works with strength
Yet shall not
    Power of radiance
Grasp
    Might of heaviness
Nor
    Might of heaviness
Penetrate
    Power of radiance
For if power of radiance grasps
    Might of heaviness
And if might of heaviness penetrates
    Power of radiance
Soul and body
    Will be bound to their ruin
In cosmic confusion.

Rudolf Steiner[164]

Wednesday / Mercury

In its orbit around the sun, as seen from the earth, Mercury describes the famous hexagram, the healing, harmonising dynamic figure which we know from the hermetic tradition as the symbol of Hermes Trismegistos, and from the Jewish tradition as the seal of Solomon.

Rudolf Steiner speaks of this in his lectures on the principles of alchemy and Rosicrucianism. The forces of our upper (light) and lower (heaviness) organisation are symbolically depicted in two triangles which interpenetrate but do not merge.[165]

We have already become familiar with these principles in the previous exercise relating to the power of radiance and the might of heaviness. Here though, rather than address the aspect of conflict, the verse concerns the healing, balancing Mercury aspect of this polarity of forces. Rudolf Steiner describes this all-encompassing, integrating principle of healing in the Easter course for young physicians.

Feel in fever's *measure*
Saturn's gift of spirit
Feel in the pulse's *count*
The *sun's* soul strength
Feel in the *weight* of matter
The forming power of the *moon*:
Then you will see in your will to heal
Also the need for healing of the *earthly* human being.

Rudolf Steiner[166]

All the forces of the four evolutionary stages of the earth itself and its creatures, starting from the great cosmic warmth body – whose radius extended from today's earth to Saturn – are characterised in their relationship with the human being on earth today.[167] Here it becomes apparent that the struggle for balance and health is not only of benefit to each individual. The "need for healing" also configures the evolutionary forces of the earth and its creatures in the cosmos which unfold through time. Human beings can learn to sense themselves as ordering, healing beings within cosmic evolution.

This meditation unites the work of physicians especially with that of nurses – the professional group for which measuring temperature, taking the pulse and monitoring weight are part of daily routine. Rudolf Steiner cites regaining a spiritual worldview that can overcome materialism as the general need for healing of human beings today. Then karmic conflicts from previous incarnations can be morally resolved rather than having to somatise themselves as illness.

Thursday / Jupiter

Jupiter is the planet of maturation, of wisdom, and of the associated pain. It remains in a single zodiac sign in the time that the sun requires to travel once through the whole zodiac. The sun's orbit relates to Jupiter as the moon's orbit does to the sun. The secret of twelve, of the seasons, of rounding off and completion is implicit in its constitution of forces.

The first meditation in the Easter course for young physicians[168] calls on us to see the whole development of the human being within the cosmos as it now is. All healing professions that approach health and illness with scientific interest and undertake anthroposophic research are united through the guidance of this meditation. This is because, for this, we need a thorough understanding of the human being and their connection with the configuring forces of the cosmos.

Only the physical body itself belongs to the earth and is attracted by it. The etheric body works entirely out of the cosmos, forming the physical body with its peripheral forces of suction. At the centre of this configuration stands the moon, whose formative power is modified by the other planets and particularly by the differing constellations of the fixed star zodiac: "And we will not get any further until astronomy – in the sense I have just explained – is reintroduced into medical science. Really most of what is said there does not mean a great deal. People juggle between one thing and another, you see, ascribing the things which occur in the human being either to external environmental conditions or to genetics.

But if you examine this in detail, it leads to nothing at all because people forget that the forming of the human being really must be derived from what arises from knowledge of the starry heavens, but in a qualitative sense, seen in accordance with its inner nature. But the most important thing with regard to such forming of the human being is the moon."[169]

The moon always exerts an influence, and the other planets support this influence.

"Behold, what is joined in the cosmos,
Thou feelest the forming of the human being."

Just as the moon is primarily connected with the human form, so the sun is connected with soul capacity, with ensoulment.

"Behold, all that moves thee in air,
Thou wilt experience the human being's ensoulment."

The capacity to spiritualise the human being can be grasped in connection with Saturn:

> "Behold, what is changed in the earthly,
> Thou wilt discern the spiritualising of the human being."[170]

Friday / Venus

Venus describes its harmonious "Pentagramma Veneris" in the heavens during a period of eight years. The form is the symbol of the upright human being, the pentagram. All physical, soul and spiritual forces work together such as to enable upright, loving human nature to come to expression at every age.

In the last lecture of the Easter course for young physicians,[171] Rudolf Steiner introduced a meditation which relates to the doctor/therapist-patient relationship and which provides the foundation for every therapeutic dialogue through to the specific therapies of biography work, psychotherapy and pastoral medical counselling. Every therapeutically-oriented encounter between human beings needs to include a sense of life as a whole, with its tendencies to illness and opportunities for healing.

The doctor/therapist works to develop imagination and inspiration in relation to the patient's etheric and astral bodies. The forces of the etheric body take care of the formation of the physical body from embryonic development through to the most advanced age. The task of the therapist is to recreate them as processes in their own soul, developing the capacity to perceive the etheric body imaginatively. The forces of the astral body, on the other hand, induce ageing with their differentiating tonal configuration, their dry, airy nature; and they exert their influence from the future back to the moment of birth. If they are sensed in a living way in their action, this leads to a grasp of the astral body through inspiration:

> Push forward infancy
> Into childhood
> And childhood
> Into youth.
> To you will appear condensed

Human etheric existence
Behind physical being –

Push back the density of old age
Into the period of human maturity
And maturity
Into youthful life.
To you will resound in cosmic tones
Human soul activity
Out of etheric life.

Rudolf Steiner[172]

"You will realise from what I have told you that guidance for meditation is not issued as a commandment but is based upon things that can be understood. Everyone instructed in meditation properly will not be treated in the authoritarian way as used to be the case in the ancient East, where both the upbringing of children and the development in old age rested upon quite different foundations from us.

When somebody is recommended meditations with us, they are given them in such a form that the person understands what they are doing with themselves. In the East the child was under the guidance of his dada. This meant that the child was taught and brought up through the way the dada lived his life. The child learned no more than he was able to learn by watching the dada. When an adult wished to make progress, he had his guru. They were dependent on the guru giving no other rule than this: thus it is – you simply need to try it.

That is the difference. What we have in our Western civilisation is that an appeal is always made to the freedom of the human being, that human beings know what they are doing. And we can also see how such inspired knowledge comes about when we have understood with common sense how physical illness and mental illness work, and when we put everything together I have told you today. For these things can be understood precisely with common sense. If we go on to understand what we should do in inner meditation, then we have reached the boundary with common sense of what we can attain. Common sense can attain everything that proceeds from anthroposophy."[173]

Saturday / Saturn

In the Pastoral Medicine Course, Rudolf Steiner summarised the physician's meditative path in its relationship with the inner path of the priest. The pastoral medicine mantra arising from this connects the work of physician and priest with the threefold divinity. Here Christ, as "Verus Mercurius", leads downwards into the realm of the elements and death to the divine Father and upwards to the Holy Spirit so as to help human beings on their ways of error towards freedom. Guilt and destiny, knowledge and transformation become comprehensible in their reciprocal influences and reveal the sources of illness and health:

> I will go the path,
> Which dissolves the elements into process
> And leads me downwards to the Father
> Who sends the illness as balance to karma.
> And leads me upwards to the Spirit
> Who guides the soul in error to attainment of freedom.
> Christ leads downwards and upwards
> Harmoniously creating spirit human being in earthly human being.
>
> *Rudolf Steiner*[174]

Working to obtain a therapeutic and educational attitude

Rudolf Steiner also included teachers/educators in the meditative path for physicians and therapists. He referred to education as "quiet healing", that is, the consistent support of healthy development. Seen in this light, education and special needs education as instruments of prevention and developmental insight also belong to the task area of physicians, nurses and therapists.

Here, above all, we are concerned with the attitude that shapes every human encounter and especially every educationally therapeutic encounter. Mystery knowledge from times when the profession of priest, physician and teacher still lay in the same hands can then be understood anew, as Steiner puts it:

> It was in ancient times,
> That there lived in the souls of initiates
> Powerfully the thought that
> By nature every human being is sick.
> And education was seen
> As a healing process
> Which, as they matured,
> Gave children the health
> To be complete human beings in life.
>
> *Rudolf Steiner*[175]

This verse harmonises with the core meditation from the Curative Education Course which Steiner introduced as the so-called point-circle meditation.[176] This exercise is at the same time the best protection for overcoming ahrimanically inspired vanity living unconsciously in the will which works counter to a therapeutically effective attitude: "Vanity is present everywhere underlying the youth movement, less so because of bad manners of any kind than for the reason that no doubt necessitates it: because the will in particular necessitates a strong development of inner capacities, vanity simply surfaces to a high degree through ahrimanic influences [...]. Hence the phenomenon we see so often: the general talk about missions and great tasks, and the disinclination to enter into the small, specific details that are required for this."[177]

Developmental steps of the Medical Section at the Goetheanum in the progression of Anthroposophic Medicine – in stages of 12 years each

Michaela Glöckler

1924

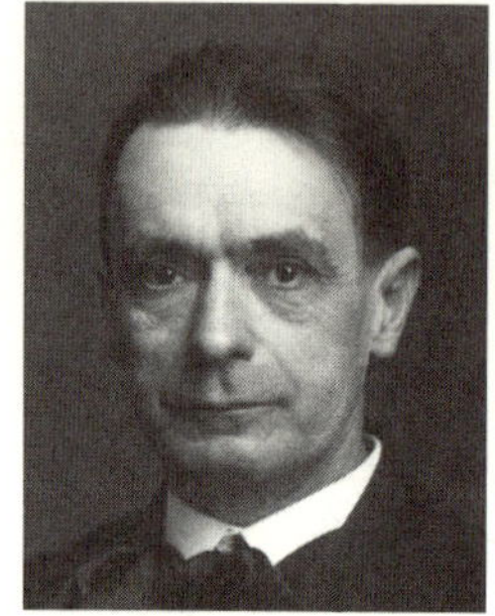
Rudolf Steiner
1861–1925

Inauguration and setting the task of working out "the medical system of anthroposophy" by Rudolf Steiner and Ita Wegman at the Christmas Conference 1923/24.

After Steiner's death, social conflicts and stresses convulse anthroposophic medicine in its further development.

Leadership of the Medical Section from 1924 to 1935:
Ita Wegman. The Anthroposophical Society is banned in Germany under the Hitler regime.

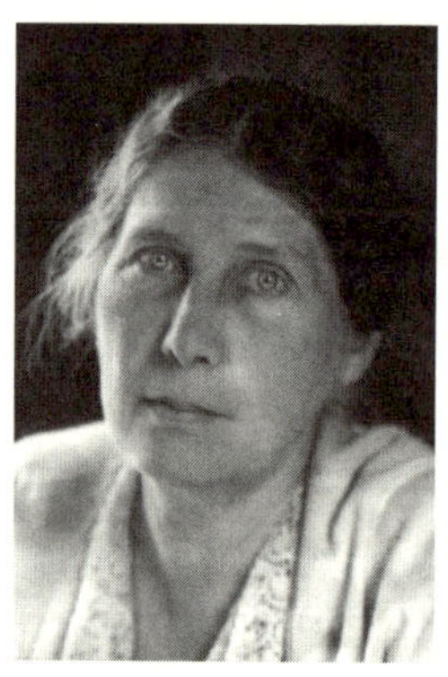
Ita Wegman
1876–1943

Interim leadership from 1935 to 1955 by the collegium:
Friedrich Husemann, Walter Bopp, Hans Zbinden, Richard Schubert

1936

Peripheralisation and spread of Anthroposophic Medicine in Europe.

Travel of Ita Wegman and clinical work in Arlesheim and Ascona.

1948

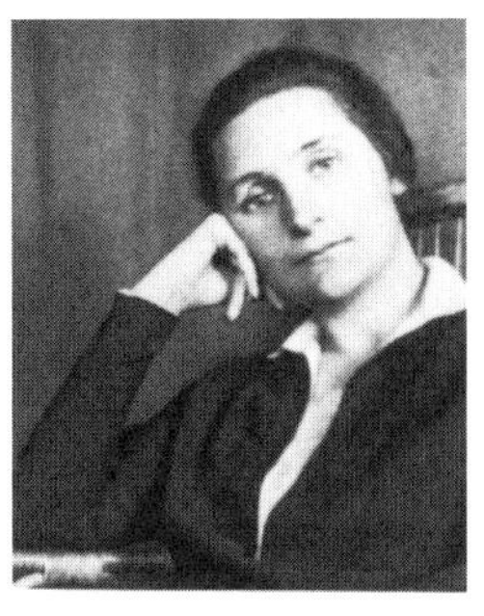
Margarete Kirchner-Bockholt
1894–1973

Attempts at social integration by various initiatives and groups to restore collaboration within the Anthroposophical Society again.

Interim leadership of the Medical Section from 1955 to 1963 by the collegium:
Hans Bleiker, Margarete Kirchner-Bockholt, Madeleine van Deventer, Gerhard Schmidt

1960

The Anthroposophical Society reforms its identity: the physician and general secretary in Holland, Willem Zeylmans van Emmichoven, reaffiliates his national society with the General Anthroposophical Society/AAG on the grounds: "Because that is what we want". Collaboration within the anthroposophic professional medical movement begins as does the new formation of the "medical core" of the Medical Section.

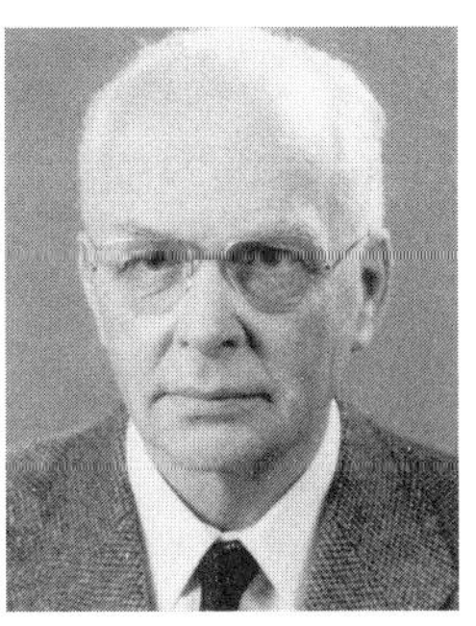
Walter Holtzapfel
1912–1994

Leadership of the Medical Section from 1963 to 1969:
Margarete Kirchner-Bockholt
Collegium: Hans Bleiker, Madeleine van Deventer, Walter Holtzapfel

Leadership of the Medical Section from 1969 to 1977:
Walter Holtzapfel
Collegium: Georg Gräflin,
Hellmut Klimm, Herbert Sieweke

1972

Institutionalisation and ensuring a legal basis for Anthroposophic Medicine in Germany: establishment of community hospitals and research establishments. Jürgen Schürholz becomes head of the newly established Commission C of the Federal Institute for Drugs and Medical Devices/BfArM covering the field of human medicine in the anthroposophic medical approach.

Leadership of the Medical Section from 1977 to 1986:
Friedrich Lorenz
Collegium: Walter Holtzapfel, Hellmut Klimm, Herbert Sieweke

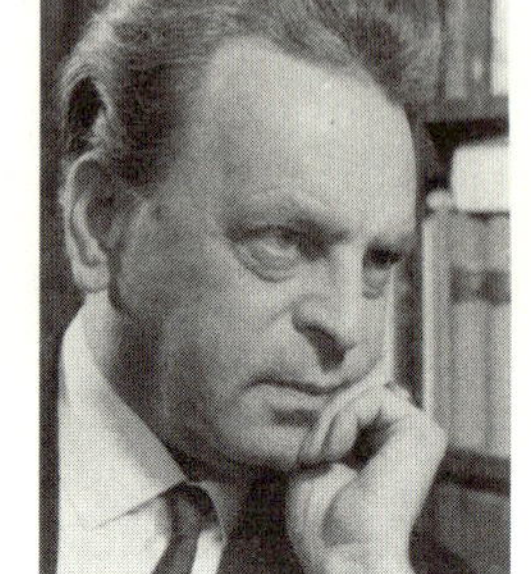

Friedrich Lorenz
1911–1987

1984

Scientific legitimisation and documentation of anthroposophic medicine in Germany and Switzerland.

Interim leadership of the Medical Section from 1986 to 1987:
Manfred Schmidt-Brabant
The collegium of the Medical Section is discharged by the executive council of the General Anthroposophical Society.

Head of the Medical Section from 1988:
Michaela Glöckler

A Section collegium working in a more representative capacity is replaced by the systematic development of international coordination and operationally active representation of the anthroposophic medical movement with its various professional groups and fields of activity.

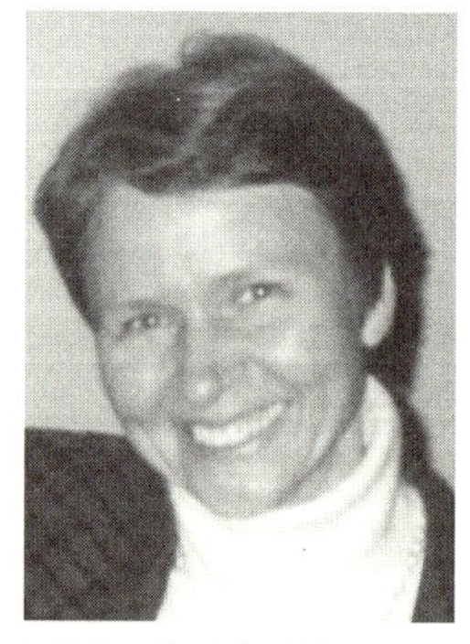

Michaela Glöckler

1996

Globalisation of Anthroposophic Medicine, EU and worldwide legitimisation processes obtain existential importance. Preparation of the first pharmacopoeia of anthroposophic medicines in the form of the Anthroposophic Pharmaceutical Codex/APC by an international group of experts.

Fundamental review of the position of anthroposophic medicine in 2000. At a "10-year conference" the representatives of anthroposophic medicine from all fields discuss what needs to be done in the coming ten years, particularly with regard to the representative books in the specialist medical fields which need to be prepared, specifically in the context of research and training, and their necessary translation into other languages. Ideas for thorough public relations work, frequently called for, take shape; well-networked websites and identity-establishing information brochures are planned and set in train. The International Coordination of Anthroposophic Medicine/IKAM takes shape as the capable leadership body of the anthroposophic medical movement.

The "blue brochures" on Anthroposophic Medicine, its medicines and therapies, conceived by Jürgen Schürholz – co-founder of the Filder Clinic and key supporter in the development of the Medical Section – and Annette Bopp, medical journalist, and published by the Medical Section, set standards, as does the new journal *Medizin Individuell*, published by Herdecke community hospital for the clinics.

The house journal of Anthroposophic Medicine *Der Merkurstab* is given a new format and layout, special issues on specific subjects are published and also translated into English.

2008 – 2020
Academisation and popularisation of Anthroposophic Medicine as a "medicine with a heart".

Realisation of the "master plan" for Anthroposophic Medicine conceived together with the Software AG foundation which aims to fund and set up chairs of anthroposophic medicine at universities. Publication of the *Vademecum of Anthroposophic Medicines*, coordinated by Georg Soldner and co-workers which is subsequently also published in English, French and Italian – other languages are in preparation. A common research base is thus created for everyday medical practice: anthroposophic physicians can now measure their own work against the latest international state of development as laid down in the medical experience set out here by 141 physicians from 15 countries and build networks for the continuous further development of Anthroposophic Medicine.

Matthias Girke conceives the "Anthromedics" project which aims to create an international platform for anthroposophic medicine in German and English, making accessible and keeping available on the Internet all important publications of anthroposophic medicine for practice-related use.

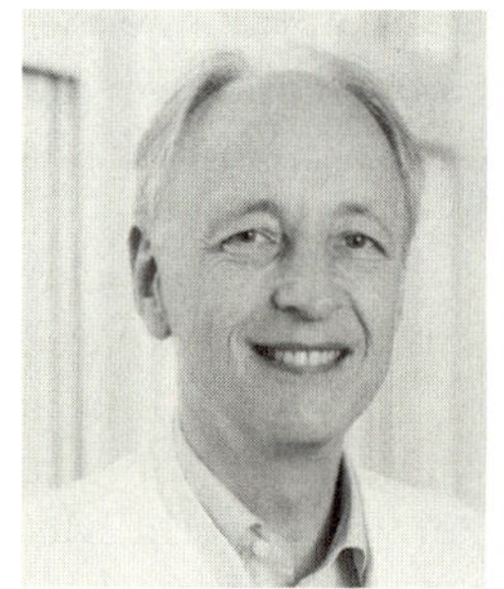

Matthias Girke

The public relations work extends its reach; the websites are given a professional makeover; CIMA is created, the first language-based, cross-country website for anthroposophic medicine in the Spanish-speaking world, as is the specialist website "Mistletoe in cancer treatment" in German and English; the patient associations cooperate to a greater extent and have a media presence.

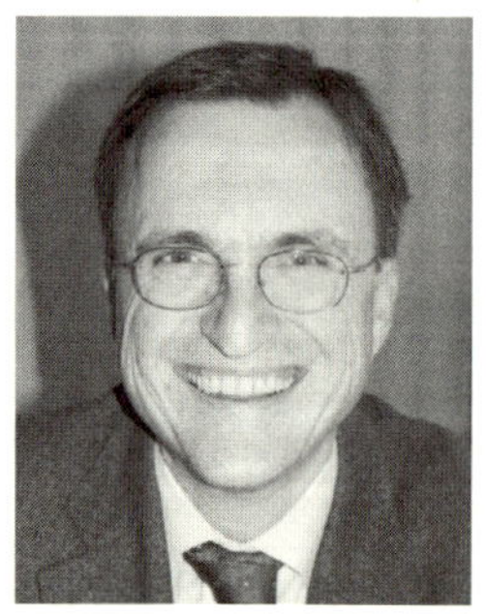

Georg Soldner

From 2016 the leadership tasks of the Medical Section are planned to be transferred to Matthias Girke and his deputy Georg Soldner.

Bibliography

Brüderlin, Markus, Gross, Ulrike (eds.): Rudolf Steiner und die Kunst der Gegenwart. Exhibition catalogue, Wolfsburg, Stuttgart 2010.

De la Houssaye, E., Heine, R. (eds.): Beiträge zur Entwicklung der Anthroposophischen Pflege 1991 – 2003; Persephone im Verlag am Goetheanum, Dornach 2006.

Domeyer, M.: Das meditative Element im Heilpädagogischen Kurs Rudolf Steiners. Meinem Freund Kurt Vierl (18.8.1924 – 26.12.2006) gewidmet. In: Seelenpflege in Heilpädagogik und Sozialtherapie, Vol. 26 (2007), No. 4, p. 4 – 18.

Glöckler, M.: Gibt es eine Prävention der Krebserkrankung? Themenheft Onkologie. Der Merkurstab 4: 416, p. 420 – 2009.

Kiersch, J.: Zur Entwicklung der Freien Hochschule für Geisteswissenschaft. Die erste Klasse. Verlag am Goetheanum, Dornach 2005, p. 50 ff., p. 201 ff., p. 288 ff.

König, K.: Vorträge zum Heilpädagogischen Kurs Rudolf Steiners. Verlag Freies Geistesleben, Stuttgart 2000.

Kries, Mateo, Vegesack, Alexander von (eds.): Rudolf Steiner – Die Alchemie des Alltags. Exhibition catalogue, Wolfsburg, Stuttgart 2010.

Kühl, J., Plato, B. von, Zimmermann, H. (eds.): Freie Hochschule für Geisteswissenschaft Goetheanum – Zur Orientierung und Einführung. Verlag am Goetheanum, Dornach 2008.

Löffler, F.: Zur Punkt-Kreis-Meditation. In: Girke, Hermann: Franz Löffler. Ein Leben für Anthroposophie und heilende Erziehung im Zeitenschicksal. Verlag am Goetheanum, Dornach 1995.

Müller-Wiedemann, H.: Menschenbild und Menschenbildung. Aufsätze und Vorträge zur Heilpädagogik, Menschenkunde und zum sozialen Leben. Verlag Freies Geistesleben, Stuttgart 1994.

Plato, B. von: Anthroposophie im 20. Jahrhundert. Verlag am Goetheanum, Dornach 2003.

Selg, P.: Die Briefkorrespondenz der "jungen Mediziner". Eine dokumentarische Studie zur Rezeption von Rudolf Steiners "Jungmediziner"-Kursen. Natura-Verlag, Dornach 2005.

Selg, P.: Die Medizin muss Ernst machen mit dem geistigen Leben. Verlag am Goetheanum, Dornach 2006.
Selg, P.: Die Wärmemeditation. Geschichtlicher Hintergrund und ideelle Beziehungen. Verlag am Goetheanum, Dornach 2005.
Selg, P.: Helene von Grunelius und Rudolf Steiners Kurse für junge Mediziner. Eine biographische Studie. Verlag am Goetheanum, Dornach 2003.
Smit, J.: Meditation und Christuserfahrung – Wege zur Verwandlung des eigenen Lebens. Freies Geistesleben, Stuttgart 2008.
Steiner, R.: Die Philosophie der Freiheit – Grundzüge einer modernen Weltanschauung (GA 4). Rudolf Steiner Verlag, Dornach 1995.
Steiner, R.: Wie erlangt man Erkenntnisse der höheren Welten? (GA 10). Rudolf Steiner Verlag, Dornach 1992.
Steiner, R.: Die Geheimwissenschaft im Umriss (GA 13). Rudolf Steiner Verlag, Dornach 1989.
Steiner, R.: Vier Mysteriendramen (GA 14). Rudolf Steiner Verlag, Dornach 1989.
Steiner, R.: Anthroposophische Leitsätze (GA 26). Rudolf Steiner Verlag, Dornach 1998.
Steiner, R., Wegman, I.: Grundlegendes für eine Erweiterung der Heilkunst nach geisteswissenschaftlichen Erkenntnissen (GA 27). Rudolf Steiner Verlag, Dornach 1991.
Steiner, R.: Wahrspruchworte (GA 40). Rudolf Steiner Verlag, Dornach 1996.
Steiner, R.: Entwicklungsgeschichtliche Unterlagen zur Bildung eines sozialen Urteils (GA 185 a). Rudolf Steiner Verlag, Dornach 2004.
Steiner, R.: Geisteswissenschaftliche Behandlung sozialer und pädagogischer Fragen (GA 192). Rudolf Steiner Verlag, Dornach 1991.
Steiner, R.: Die Brücke zwischen der Weltgeistigkeit und dem Physischen des Menschen. Die Suche nach der neuen Isis, der göttlichen Sophia (GA 202). Rudolf Steiner Verlag, Dornach 1993.
Steiner, R.: Das Miterleben des Jahreslaufes in vier kosmischen Imaginationen (GA 229). Rudolf Steiner Verlag, Dornach 1999.
Steiner, R.: Mysteriengestaltungen (GA 232). Rudolf Steiner Verlag, Dornach 1998.
Steiner, R.: Die Weltgeschichte in anthroposophischer Beleuchtung und als Grundlage der Erkenntnis des Menschengeistes (GA 233). Rudolf Steiner Verlag, Dornach 1991.

Steiner, R.: Mysterienstätten des Mittelalters (GA 233 a). Rudolf Steiner Verlag, Dornach 1991.

Steiner, R.: Die Weihnachtstagung zur Begründung der Allgemeinen Anthroposophischen Gesellschaft 1923/1924 (GA 260). Rudolf Steiner Verlag, Dornach 1994.

Steiner, R.: Die Konstitution der Allgemeinen Anthroposophischen Gesellschaft und der Freien Hochschule für Geisteswissenschaft (GA 260 a). Rudolf Steiner Verlag, Dornach 1987.

Steiner, R.: Zur Geschichte und aus den Inhalten der ersten Abteilung der Esoterischen Schule 1904–1924, Briefe, Rundbriefe, Dokumente und Vorträge (GA 264). Rudolf Steiner Verlag, Dornach 1996.

Steiner, R.: Zur Geschichte und aus den Inhalten der erkenntniskultischen Abteilung der Esoterischen Schule von 1904 bis 1914 (GA 265). Rudolf Steiner Verlag, Dornach 1987.

Steiner, R.: Mantrische Sprüche. Seelenübungen Band II (GA 268). Rudolf Steiner Verlag, Dornach 1999.

Steiner, R.: Eurythmie. Die Offenbarung der sprechenden Seele (GA 277). Rudolf Steiner Verlag, Dornach 1999.

Steiner, R.: Eurythmie als sichtbarer Gesang (GA 278). Rudolf Steiner Verlag, Dornach 2001.

Steiner, R.: Eurythmie als sichtbare Sprache (GA 279). Rudolf Steiner Verlag, Dornach 1990.

Steiner, R.: Wege zu einem neuen Baustil (GA 286). Rudolf Steiner Verlag, Dornach 1982.

Steiner, R.: Geisteswissenschaft und Medizin (GA 312). Rudolf Steiner Verlag, Dornach 1999.

Steiner, R.: Geisteswissenschaftliche Gesichtspunkte zur Therapie (GA 313). Rudolf Steiner Verlag, Dornach 2001.

Steiner, R.: Physiologisch-Therapeutisches auf Grundlage der Geisteswissenschaft (GA 314). Rudolf Steiner Verlag, Dornach 1989.

Steiner, R.: Heileurythmie (GA 315). Rudolf Steiner Verlag, Dornach 2003.

Steiner, R.: Meditative Betrachtungen und Anleitungen zur Vertiefung der Heilkunst (GA 316). Rudolf Steiner Verlag, Dornach 2008.

Steiner, R.: Heilpädagogischer Kurs (GA 317). Rudolf Steiner Verlag, Dornach 1995.

Steiner, R.: Das Zusammenwirken von Ärzten und Seelsorgern – Pastoral-Medizinischer Kurs (GA 318). Rudolf Steiner Verlag, Dornach 1994.

Steiner, R.: Anthroposophische Menschenerkenntnis und Medizin (GA 319). Rudolf Steiner Verlag, Dornach 1994.
Steiner, R.: Geisteswissenschaftliche Grundlagen zum Gedeihen der Landwirtschaft (GA 327). Rudolf Steiner Verlag, Dornach 1999.
Steiner, R.: Vom Einheitsstaat zum dreigliedrigen sozialen Organismus (GA 334). Rudolf Steiner Verlag, Dornach 1983.
Steiner, R.: Die Krisis der Gegenwart und der Weg zu gesundem Denken (GA 335). Rudolf Steiner Verlag, Dornach 2005.
Steiner, R.: Soziale Ideen – Soziale Wirklichkeit – Soziale Praxis (GA 337 b). Rudolf Steiner Verlag, Dornach 1999.
Steiner, R.: Das Geheimnis der Wunde – Aufzeichnungen zum Samariterkurs (Beiträge zur Rudolf Steiner Gesamtausgabe, Heft 108). Rudolf Steiner Verlag, Dornach 1992.
Vademecum Anthroposophische Arzneimittel (publ.: Gesellschaft Anthroposophischer Ärzte in Deutschland, Medizinische Sektion am Goetheanum): Supplement Merkurstab 2008, Filderstadt 2008.
Vademecum of Anthroposophic Medicines (Published by: Medical Section of the School of Spiritual Science, International Federation of Anthroposophic Medical Associations [IVAA], Association of Anthroposophic Physicians in Germany [GAÄD]). Supplement: Der Merkurstab 4. Journal of Anthroposophic Medicine. Volume 62, 2009.
Wiesberger, H.: Rudolf Steiners esoterische Lehrtätigkeit. Rudolf Steiner Verlag, Dornach 1997.
Zeylmans van Emmichoven, J. E.: Wer war Ita Wegman (Volume 1). Edition Georgenberg, Heidelberg 1999. Rudolf Steiners Zusammenarbeit mit Ita Wegman. Verlag am Goetheanum, Dornach 2013.
Zeylmans van Emmichoven, J. E.: Die Erkraftung des Herzens. Eine Mysterienschulung der Gegenwart. Edited by Cordula Zeylmans van Emmichoven. Verlag des Ita Wegman Instituts, Arlesheim 2009.
Zuck, R.: Das Recht der Anthroposophischen Medizin. Nomos, Baden-Baden 2007.

Finances of the Medical Section

Finding the financial resources needed by the School of Spiritual Science, and with it the Medical Section, has become an existential challenge today. This is all the more so as fundamentally there is barely adequate financial compensation for the services provided by Anthroposophic Medicine and there are thus small surpluses but rarely is there an abundance.

A voluntary and regular financial contribution from the co-workers of the anthroposophic medical movement to safeguard the work of the Section leadership and its most immediate staff would represent a first necessary step for sustainably assuring the worldwide impulses of Anthroposophic Medicine through its ideas, its social networks and public representation.

In the summer of 2014, Michaela Glöckler turned to the co-workers of the anthroposophic medical movement with the following Newsletter. As the International Coordination Group (IKAM) we expressly support this impulse.

Newsletter of the Medical Section, Summer 2014

That good may become
What from our hearts we found,
and from our heads
we direct with single purpose.
Rudolf Steiner

Dear friends,

This newsletter is devoted to the finances of the Medical Section at the Goetheanum which this year celebrates its ninetieth birthday. It was founded at Christmas 1923 as part of the School of Spiritual Science. It received its esoteric content through the Young Physicians' Course as well as the Agricultural Course and Curative Education Course, which Rudolf Steiner gave in 1924; the Pastoral Medicine Course during September 1924 provided the basis for a spiritual community for physicians.

Steiner's idea was that the membership of the Anthroposophical Society would increasingly be in a position to finance the School. He reasoned that this was the only way to guarantee a truly free spiritual life. Because if sponsors, foundations and companies give money, they understandably also have an interest in supporting specific projects and activities with that money which accord with their own thinking and work. In contrast, the School with its sections was to be free to conduct research and also take up initiatives whose relevance might perhaps only become clear years later. It was also to have the opportunity to invest time and strength so that people could encounter one another, maintain social connections, and there could be an awareness of initiatives and people worldwide who wanted to put anthroposophy into practice – often under difficult circumstances. This was to be allowed for even if it is not always possible to negotiate a price for everything before or after the event.

Rudolf Steiner's brilliant idea requires a metamorphosis in the present time as the membership of the Anthroposophical

Society is not currently growing and we are very grateful that it nevertheless manages to care for and maintain the Goetheanum and its operations as well as the building itself and the surrounding land with its particular wealth of plants and insects.

What is thus needed, is a group of people and institutions who are willing to make a firm commitment to provide the necessary financial resources which are required for the various sections of the School so that they can continue to function. For the Medical Section this means that the salary of the Section head, the head's assistant, a half-time secretariat post and a research associate, as well as the associated office and incidental expenses, have to be secured. This administrative pillar should comprise about one third of the annual budget. This is not much in comparison to other nonprofit organisations, associations and higher education institutions but would safeguard the existence of the sections and their ability to do their work. All other research activity, training and advanced training, conferences and events as well as other projects could then be undertaken as the income-generating activity of each section itself or with the help of project financing from foundations or with sponsorship money.

The current situation is that, together with the free use of the Section premises, only five percent of the annual budget of the Medical Section is assured by the Anthroposophical Society. This means in concrete terms that as Section head I have to take care myself of a part of my salary through lecture fees etc., and that assuring the salaries of the Section staff each year represents a real entrepreneurial challenge. That is not a healthy situation. Hence we have repeatedly made an effort in recent years to place the work of the Section on a more healthy financial footing. Thus one consideration was to organise the Medical Section like an umbrella organisation with fixed membership fees, annual general meetings, statements of accounts etc. But it quickly became clear that democratic usages would endanger the free spiritual life just as much as being tied to the interests of sponsors or firms as described above.

In this situation I had a meeting on the sidelines of an IPMT advanced training week for Anthroposophic Medicine with Harald Matthes, physician-in-charge at the Havelhöhe community hospital, Berlin, and a member of the Weleda board of directors.

Not only did he very quickly understand the need for action but he also offered to hold discussions with AM institutions and associations as to whether they would be prepared to give a free regular undertaking of funding for the administrative pillar of the Medical Section. This is well on the way to being realised for the first time in 2014, for which we are exceedingly grateful.

But the undertakings given so far are not sufficient to cover the required third of the Section budget. That is why today I turn to all of you with a huge request, namely whether it would not be possible to make a "voluntary co-worker contribution" to the Medical Section this year which might, for example, correspond to the fee for an hour of patient time. Already almost 100 of the 20,000 co-workers and friends worldwide do this each year. Each single person who makes such a commitment counts! The following link can be used to put such a supportive intention into practice immediately: http://www.medsektion-goetheanum.org/projekte/ jetztspenden/.

If we succeeded making this financial foundation a reality, the Medical Section would definitively be out of its pioneering phase and could develop into the twenty-first century in a healthy way. It is needed more than ever as a free spiritual space for encounter and work. It has no interests of its own, no "country", no "power" – which means that it is also easily forgotten. But with it, all the things we do for AM worldwide work "more easily" in a mysterious way, as if "borne by the spirit". Because it maintains the spiritual connection with the origins of Anthroposophic Medicine, tries to help where needed with the overview and competence it has developed over decades, and wishes to bear living testimony to Rudolf Steiner's work in the social sphere and its possibility of initiating spiritual and selflessly active, free working communities. All of us can help in this and feel ourselves to be part of the whole.

In this spirit I today send not only warm but also very hopeful greetings – also on behalf of Stefan Langhammer who is responsible for the financial management of the Section.

Yours
Michaela Glöckler

For donations from Switzerland:

Allgemeine Anthroposophische Gesellschaft, Medizinische Sektion,
Raiffeisenbank Dornach, Account 10060.56
Clearing: 80939, Postal account 40-9606-4
IBAN: CH36 8093 9000 0010 0605 6
BIC: RAIFCH22

For Donations from Germany or other countries:

Medizinische Sektion bei der Förderstiftung AM,
Volksbank Dreiländereck, Account 970760
Bank sort code: 683 900 00
IBAN: DE92 6839 0000 0000 9707 60
BIC: VOLODE66

Our address:

Medizinische Sektion am Goetheanum
Postfach
4143 Dornach 1, Switzerland
Tel +41(61) 706 42 90
Fax +41 (61) 706 42 91
sekretariat@medsektion-goetheanum.ch
www.medsektion-goetheanum.org

Picture Credits

With kind permission

of the Rudolf Steiner Nachlassverwaltung: page 30 (diagram about School) and page 147 (blackboard drawing of point-circle meditation),

of the Verlag am Goetheanum: page 45 (Representative of Humanity)

and of the Ita Wegman Archive: page 220 (photo of Ita Wegman).

The image rights in the remaining pictures reside with the Medical Section at the Goetheanum.

Notes

1 Steiner, M.: Vorwort zur 1. Auflage 1944. In: Steiner, R.: Die Weihnachtstagung zur Begründung der Allgemeinen Anthroposophischen Gesellschaft 1923/1924. Rudolf Steiner Verlag, Dornach 1994, p. 13 ff.

2 Kühl, J., Plato, B. von, Zimmermann, H. (eds.): Freie Hochschule für Geisteswissenschaft am Goetheanum – Zur Orientierung und Einführung. Verlag am Goetheanum, Dornach 2008.

3 See also: The System of Anthroposophic Medicine: https://www. ivaa.info/fileadmin/editor/file/The_system_of_Anthroposophic_Medicine_2014.pdf and publications on Anthroposophic Medicine: https://www.medsektion-goetheanum.org/en/home/publications/.

4 Steiner, R.: Die Weihnachtstagung zur Begründung der Allgemeinen Anthroposophischen Gesellschaft 1923/1924 (GA 260). Rudolf Steiner Verlag, Dornach 1994, p. 142, Continuation of the foundation meeting, Dornach, 28. 12. 1923.

5 Ibid. p. 20.

6 Zuck, R.: Das Recht der Anthroposophischen Medizin. Nomos Verlag, Baden-Baden 2012.

7 Steiner, R.: Allgemeine Menschenkunde als Grundlage der Pädagogik (GA 293). Rudolf Steiner Verlag, Dornach 1992, First lecture of 21 August 1919.

8 Steiner, R.: Meditative Betrachtungen und Anleitungen zur Vertiefung der Heilkunst (GA 316). Rudolf Steiner Verlag, Dornach 2008, p. 102, Seventh lecture, 8 January 1924.

9 See Steiner, R.: Esoterische Unterweisungen für die erste Klasse der Freien Hochschule für Geisteswissenschaft am Goetheanum (GA 270 I–IV). Rudolf Steiner Verlag, Dornach 2008.

10 Aus den Inhalten der esoterischen Stunden. Gedächtnisaufzeichnungen von Teilnehmern und Meditationstexte nach Niederschriften Rudolf Steiners. Volume III: 1913 and 1914, 1920–1923 (GA 266c). Rudolf Steiner Verlag, Dornach 1998, p. 436.

11 See note 5, Opening lecture of 24 December 1923, p. 35.

12 Steiner, R.: Die Konstitution der Allgemeinen Anthroposophischen Gesellschaft und der Freien Hochschule für Geisteswissenschaft (GA 260a). Rudolf Steiner Verlag, Dornach 1987, p. 131 ff., Nachrichtenblatt, 3 February 1924.

13 Steiner, R.: Theosophie. Einführung in übersinnliche Welterkenntnis und Menschenbestimmung (GA 9). Rudolf Steiner Verlag, Dornach 1978, p. 176.

14 Steiner, R.: Geisteswissenschaftliche Behandlung sozialer und pädagogischer Fragen (GA 192). Rudolf Steiner Verlag, Dornach 1991, p. 61 ff., Third lecture, Stuttgart, 1 May 1919.
15 See also Smit, J.: Meditation und Christuserfahrung – Wege zur Verwandlung des eigenen Lebens. Verlag Freies Geistesleben, Stuttg. 2008.
16 Steiner, R.: Wie erlangt man Erkenntnisse der höheren Welten? (GA 10). Rudolf Steiner Verlag, Dornach 1992, p. 75 ff.
17 Steiner, R.: Die Philosophie der Freiheit – Grundzüge einer modernen Weltanschauung (GA 4). Rudolf Steiner Verlag, Dornach 1995, p. 145 ff.
18 Steiner, R.: Die Weihnachtstagung zur Begründung der Allgemeinen Anthroposophischen Gesellschaft 1923/1924 (GA 260). Rudolf Steiner Verlag, Dornach 1994, p. 113, Continuation of the foundation meeting, Dornach, 27 December 1923.
19 See previous note, p. 48 ff., Statute proposal, Dornach, 24 December 1923.
20 Ibid. p. 43.
21 Ibid. p. 161.
22 See printed manuscript of the School of Spiritual Science. Goetheanum, Dornach 2002, p. 29, p. 37, p. 47.
23 Ibid. p. 40, p. 28, p. 34, p. 64.
24 Ibid. p. 62.
25 Steiner, R.: Briefe an die Mitglieder 1924. Rudolf Steiner Verlag, Dornach 1987.
26 Ibid., Lecture of 5 September 1924.
27 Given personally, printed source unknown.
28 Steiner, R.: Anthroposophische Menschenerkenntnis und Medizin (GA 319), lecture of 28 August 1923. Rudolf Steiner Verlag, Dornach 1982.
29 Ibid., Lecture of 9 January 1924.
30 Zeylmans van Emmichoven, J. E.: Wer war Ita Wegman. Volume 2. Natura Verlag, Arlesheim 2000, p. 216–217 and Glöckler, M.: Medizin an der Schwelle. Verlag am Goetheanum, Dornach 1993, p. 48 f.
31 From: Glöckler, M.: Zur Erneuerung des Mysterienwesens. In: Glöckler, M. (ed.): Medizin an der Schwelle. Verlag am Goetheanum, Dornach 1992, p. 48 ff.
32 Selg, P.: Die Briefkorrespondenz der «jungen Mediziner». Eine dokumentarische Studie zur Rezeption von Rudolf Steiners «Jungmediziner»-Kurs. Verlag am Goetheanum, Dornach 2005.
33 Steiner, R.: Ansprache an die Mediziner vom 18. September 1924. In: Das Zusammenwirken von Ärzten und Seelsorgern. Pastoral-Medizinischer Kurs (GA 318). Rudolf Steiner Verlag, Dornach 1994, p. 164 ff.
34 Steiner, R.: Es sprach Merkur-Raphael. In: Mantrische Sprüche (GA 268). Rudolf Steiner Verlag, Dornach 1999, p. 309.

35 Wiesberger, H.: Rudolf Steiners esoterische Lehrtätigkeit. Rudolf Steiner Verlag, Dornach 1997, p. 23, p. 306 and Kiersch, J.: Zur Entwicklung der Freien Hochschule für Geisteswissenschaft. Die erste Klasse. Verlag am Goetheanum, Dornach 2005, p. 50 ff., p. 201 ff., p. 288 ff.

36 Steiner, R.: Zur Geschichte und aus den Inhalten der ersten Abteilung der Esoterischen Schule 1904–1924, Briefe, Rundbriefe, Dokumente und Vorträge (GA 264). Rudolf Steiner Verlag, Dornach 1996, p. 421 ff. Address, Berlin, 15 December 1911.

37 von Plato, B. (ed.): Anthroposophie im 20. Jahrhundert. Verlag am Goetheanum. Dornach 2003, p. 1009 ff. and Sease, V.: Rudolf Steiners Versuch einer Stiftung für theosophische Art und Kunst – 15 December 1911. Verlag am Goetheanum, Dornach 2011.

38 Steiner, R.: Vier Mysteriendramen (GA 14). Rudolf Steiner Verlag, Dornach 1989.

39 Steiner, R.: Die Konstitution der Allgemeinen Anthroposophischen Gesellschaft und der Freien Hochschule für Geisteswissenschaft (GA 260 a). Rudolf Steiner Verlag, Dornach 1987, p. 25 ff. Letters to Members.

40 See also Steiner, R.: Esoterische Betrachtungen karmischer Zusammenhänge (GA 237). Rudolf Steiner Verlag, Dornach 1991, p. 120 ff., Lecture of 1 August 1924.

41 Steiner, R.: Geisteswissenschaft, Evangelium und Menschheitszukunft. In: Die Apokalypse des Johannes (GA 104). Rudolf Steiner Verlag, Dornach 2006.

42 Steiner, R.: Wie erlangt man Erkenntnisse der höheren Welten? (GA 10). Rudolf Steiner Verlag, Dornach 1992, p. 75 ff.

43 Steiner, R.: Die Weihnachtstagung zur Begründung der Allgemeinen Anthroposophischen Gesellschaft 1923/1924 (GA 260). Rudolf Steiner Verlag, Dornach 1994, p. 278, Lecture and parting words by Rudolf Steiner, Dornach, 1 January 1924.

44 Steiner, R.: Meditative Betrachtungen und Anleitungen zur Vertiefung der Heilkunst (GA 316). Rudolf Steiner Verlag, Dornach 2008. Seventh lecture, Dornach, 8 January 1924, p. 103 ff.

45 Shown using the example of cancer in Glöckler, M.: Gibt es eine Prävention der Krebserkrankung? Themenheft Onkologie. Der Merkurstab 4: 416, p. 420 – 2009.

46 Steiner, R.: Mantrische Sprüche. Seelenübungen Volume II (GA 268). Rudolf Steiner Verlag, Dornach 1999, p. 304, Notebook, January 1924.

47 See also Society of Anthroposophic Physicians in Germany, Medical Section at the Goetheanum (eds.): Vademecum Anthroposophische Arzneimittel. Supplement Merkurstab, Filderstadt ^{3}2013.

48 Walter Holtzapfel, head of the Medical Section from 1969 to 1977, developed this approach further in his book: Auf dem Wege zum Hygienischen Okkultismus. Verlag am Goetheanum, Dornach 2008.

49 Steiner, R.: Meditative Betrachtungen und Anleitungen zur Vertiefung der Heilkunst (GA 316). Rudolf Steiner Verlag, Dornach 2008, p. 223, First newsletter for physicians, 11 March 1924. See also Glöckler, M. (ed.): Das Schulkind – gemeinsame Aufgaben von Arzt und Lehrer. Verlag am Goetheanum, Dornach 1998 and Glöckler, M.; Langhammer, S.; Wiechert, C. (ed.): Gesundheit durch Erziehung. Medizinische Sektion am Goetheanum, Dornach 2006.
50 Steiner, R.: Die Weihnachtstagung zur Begründung der Allgemeinen Anthroposophischen Gesellschaft 1923/1924 (GA 260). Rudolf Steiner Verlag, Dornach 1994, p. 287, Words of thanks from the members and concluding words by Rudolf Steiner, Dornach, 1 January 1924.
51 Galatians 2:20, quoted from the King James Bible.
52 The exhibitions in Wolfsburg and Stuttgart in 2010 illustrate Steiner's influence on art in a particularly impressive way: see Brüderlin, M.; Gross, U. (eds.): Rudolf Steiner und die Kunst der Gegenwart. Exhibition catalogue, Wolfsburg, Stuttgart 2010 and Kries, M.; von Vegesack, A. (eds.): Rudolf Steiner – Die Alchemie des Alltags. Exhibition catalogue, Wolfsburg, Stuttgart 2010.
53 Steiner, R.: Wege zu einem neuen Baustil (GA 286). Rudolf Steiner Verlag, Dornach 1982, p. 74, Second lecture, Dornach, 17 June 1914.
54 Steiner, R.: Soziale Ideen – Soziale Wirklichkeit – Soziale Praxis (GA 337b). Rudolf Steiner Verlag, Dornach 1999, p. 242, Second evening of questions, Dornach, 12 October 1920.
55 Steiner, R.: Die Weihnachtstagung zur Begründung der Allgemeinen Anthroposophischen Gesellschaft 1923/1924 (GA 260). Rudolf Steiner Verlag, Dornach 1994, p. 36, Opening lecture, 24 December 1923.
56 Ibid. p. 284, Lecture and parting words by Rudolf Steiner. Dornach, 1 January 1924.
57 Steiner, R.: Meditative Betrachtungen und Anleitungen zur Vertiefung der Heilkunst (GA 316). Rudolf Steiner Verlag, Dornach 2008, p. 220, Fifth lecture, 25 April 1924.
58 See also Furst, B.: The Heart and Circulation. An Integrative Model. Springer, London 2014.
59 Lucifer/Diabolos and Ahriman/Satanas are the two demonic figures whom Goethe put on the stage under the name of Mephisto in *Faust* 1 and 2. Rudolf Steiner did this in his four Mystery Dramas.
60 Steiner, R.: Vom Einheitsstaat zum dreigliedrigen sozialen Organismus (GA 334). Rudolf Steiner Verlag, Dornach 1983, p. 242, First lecture, Basel, 4 May 1920.
61 Steiner, R.: Soziale Ideen – Soziale Wirklichkeit – Soziale Praxis (GA 337b). Rudolf Steiner Verlag, Dornach 1999, p. 52, Third discussion evening, Dornach, 9 August 1920.
62 Steiner, R.: Die Konstitution der Allgemeinen Anthroposophischen Gesellschaft und der Freien Hochschule für Geisteswissenschaft (GA

260a). Rudolf Steiner Verlag, Dornach 1987, p. 123, The School of Spiritual Science within the constitution of the Anthroposophical Society, its division into sections, Dornach, 30 January 1924.

63 See Steiner, R.: Wie erlangt man Erkenntnisse der höheren Welten? (GA 10). Rudolf Steiner Verlag, Dornach 1992.

64 Steiner, R.: Die Weihnachtstagung zur Begründung der Allgemeinen Anthroposophischen Gesellschaft 1923/1924 (GA 260). Rudolf Steiner Verlag, Dornach 1994, p. 48 ff., Opening lecture, Dornach, 24 December 1923.

65 Ibid. p. 49, Article 2 of the statutes of the Anthroposophical Society.

66 Steiner, R.: Die Geheimwissenschaft im Umriss (GA 13). Rudolf Steiner Verlag, Dornach 1989, p. 314/15.

67 Ibid. p. 396.

68 Steiner, R.: Wie erlangt man Erkenntnisse der höheren Welten? (GA 10). Rudolf Steiner Verlag, Dornach 1992, p. 215.

69 Ibid. p. 214.

70 Steiner, R.: Kosmische und menschliche Geschichte (GA 171). Rudolf Steiner Verlag, Dornach 1984, p. 137.

71 Steiner, R.: Die Geheimwissenschaft im Umriss (GA 13). Rudolf Steiner Verlag, Dornach 1989, p. 406 f.

72 Steiner, R.: Die Weihnachtstagung zur Begründung der Allgemeinen Anthroposophischen Gesellschaft 1923/1924 (GA 260). Rudolf Steiner Verlag, Dornach 1994, p. 48 ff., Opening lecture, Dornach, 24 December 1923.

73 Klett, M.: Zur Aufgabe der Sektionen der Freien Hochschule für Geisteswissenschaft am Goetheanum. Section for Agriculture, Dornach 2014.

74 Steiner, R.: Die Weihnachtstagung zur Begründung der Allgemeinen Anthroposophischen Gesellschaft 1923/1924 (GA 260). Rudolf Steiner Verlag, Dornach 1994, p. 80.

75 Ibid. p. 140 and p. 161.

76 A selection of his works: Friedrich Glasl: Konfliktmanagement. Ein Handbuch für Führungskräfte, Beraterinnen und Berater. Haupt-Verlag, Bern 2009. Id., Konfliktfähigkeit statt Streitlust oder Konfliktscheu. Verlag am Goetheanum, Dornach 2010. Id., Das Unternehmen der Zukunft. Moralische Intuition in der Gestaltung von Organisationen. Verlag Freies Geistesleben, Stuttgart 1999. Id., Konflikt, Krise, Katharsis. Verlag Freies Geistesleben, Stuttgart 2008.

77 Steiner, R.: Die Philosophie der Freiheit (GA 4). Rudolf Steiner Verlag, Dornach 1995, p. 158.

78 Cf. also p. 49 f. where reference was already made to the principle of individuality and the Goetheanum leadership was mentioned.

79 Cf. p. 49.

80 Steiner, R.: Heilpädagogischer Kurs (GA 317). Rudolf Steiner Verlag, Dornach 1995, p. 187.

81 See p. 60.
82 Cf. Steiner, R.: Esoterische Betrachtungen karmischer Zusammenhänge. Dritter Band. Die karmischen Zusammenhänge der anthroposophischen Bewegung (GA 237). Rudolf Steiner Verlag, Dornach 1991, Lecture of 8 July 1924.
83 Steiner, R.: Die Weihnachtstagung zur Begründung der Allgemeinen Anthroposophischen Gesellschaft 1923/1924 (GA 260). 26.12.1923. Rudolf Steiner Verlag, Dornach 1994.
84 Steiner, R.: Geisteswissenschaft und Medizin (GA 312). Rudolf Steiner Verlag, Dornach 1999. Id.: Geisteswissenschaftliche Gesichtspunkte zur Therapie (GA 313). Rudolf Steiner Verlag, Dornach 2011. Id.: Physiologisch-Therapeutisches auf Grundlage der Geisteswissenschaft (GA 314). Rudolf Steiner Verlag, Dornach 1989. Id.: Meditative Betrachtungen und Anleitungen zur Vertiefung der Heilkunst (GA 316). Rudolf Steiner Verlag, Dornach 2008.
85 Steiner, R.: Wahrspruchworte (GA 40). Rudolf Steiner Verlag, Dornach 1981, p. 116.
86 Steiner, R.: Meditative Betrachtungen und Anleitungen zur Vertiefung der Heilkunst (GA 316). Rudolf Steiner Verlag, Dornach 2008.
87 Ibid.
88 Ibid. p. 69–70.
89 Ibid. p. 128–129.
90 Steiner, R.: Mantrische Sprüche. Seelenübungen Band II (GA 268). Rudolf Steiner Verlag, Dornach 1999, p. 296 ff. To Helene von Grunelius for the physicians, autumn 1923.
91 Ibid. p. 27.
92 Ibid.
93 Steiner, R.: Meditative Betrachtungen und Anleitungen zur Vertiefung der Heilkunst (GA 316). Rudolf Steiner Verlag, Dornach 2008, p. 70 f., Fourth lecture, 5 January 1924. See the text of the mantra also in GA 268.
94 Neumann, M.; Edelhäuser, F., Tauschel, D. et al.: Empathy Decline and Its Reasons: A Systematic Review of Studies With Medical Students and Residents. Academic Medicine 86: p. 996 – 1009, 2011.
95 Steiner, R.: Meditative Betrachtungen und Anleitungen zur Vertiefung der Heilkunst (GA 316). Rudolf Steiner Verlag, Dornach 2008, p. 70.
96 Ibid. p. 138, Eighth lecture, Dornach, 9 January 1924.
97 Ibid. p. 129.
98 Ibid. p. 133.
99 Ibid. p. 223, First newsletter for physicians, 11 March 1924.
100 Ibid. p. 223.
101 Ibid. p. 172.
102 Ibid.
103 Ibid. p. 173.

104 Ibid. p. 200 ff., Fourth lecture, Dornach, 24 April 1924.
105 Ibid. p. 173.
106 Ibid. p. 200.
107 Ibid. p. 213 f.
108 Ibid. p. 213.
109 Ibid. p. 214.
110 Steiner, R.: Faksimile in de la Houssaye, E.; Heine, R.: Beiträge zur Entwicklung der Anthroposophischen Pflege; Persephone, Dornach 2005.
111 Steiner, R.: Mantrische Sprüche. Seelenübungen Band II (GA 268). Rudolf Steiner Verlag, Dornach 1999, p. 115.
112 Ibid.
113 Ibid. p. 195
114 Ibid. p. 196.
115 Steiner, R.: Meditative Betrachtungen und Anleitungen zur Vertiefung der Heilkunst (GA 316). Rudolf Steiner Verlag, Dornach 2008, p. 200, Fourth lecture, Dornach, 24 April 1924.
116 Reiner, J. (ed.): In der Nacht sind wir zwei Menschen. Arbeitseinblicke in die anthroposophische Psychotherapie. Verlag Freies Geistesleben, Stuttgart 2012.
117 Ibid., Johannes Reiner in the foreword.
118 Steiner, R.: Mantrische Sprüche. Seelenübungen Band II (GA 268). Rudolf Steiner Verlag, Dornach 1999, p. 306.
119 Steiner, R.: Meditative Betrachtungen und Anleitungen zur Vertiefung der Heilkunst (GA 316). Rudolf Steiner Verlag, Dornach 2008, p. 138.
120 Steiner, R.: Das Zusammenwirken von Ärzten und Seelsorgern. Pastoral-Medizinischer Kurs (GA 318). Rudolf Steiner Verlag, Dornach 1994, p. 163.
121 Steiner, R.: Seelenübungen mit Wort- und Sinnbild-Meditationen (GA 267). Rudolf Steiner Verlag, Dornach 2001, p. 213.
122 Steiner, R.: Heilpädagogischer Kurs (GA 317). Rudolf Steiner Verlag, Dornach 1995.
123 Steiner, R.: Eurythmie als sichtbare Sprache (GA 279). Fourteenth lecture of 11 July 1924. Rudolf Steiner Verlag, Dornach 1990.
124 Ibid. p. 238.
125 Steiner, R.: Eurythmie als sichtbarer Gesang (GA 278). Rudolf Steiner Verlag, Dornach 2001, p. 83.
126 Steiner, R.: Mysterienstätten des Mittelalters. Rosenkreuzertum und modernes Einweihungsprinzip (GA 233a). Rudolf Steiner Verlag, Dornach 1991, p. 71.
127 Steiner, R.: Meditative Betrachtungen und Anleitungen zur Vertiefung der Heilkunst (GA 316). Rudolf Steiner Verlag, Dornach 2008, p. 133.
128 Ibid., Christmas course, Eighth lecture of 9 January 1924.
129 Ibid., Easter course, Second lecture of 22 April 1924.

130 Ibid., Third lecture of 23 April 1924.
131 Ibid.
132 Ibid., see complete mantra on p. 173.
133 Steiner, R.: Mantrische Sprüche. Seelenübungen Band II (GA 268). Rudolf Steiner Verlag, Dornach 1999, p. 268 ff.
134 Steiner, R.: Meditative Betrachtungen und Anleitungen zur Vertiefung der Heilkunst (GA 316). Rudolf Steiner Verlag, Dornach 2008, p. 138, Eighth lecture, Dornach, 9 January 1924.
135 Steiner, R.: Methodik und Wesen der Sprachgestaltung. Rudolf Steiner Verlag, Dornach 1983, p. 21.
136 Steiner, R.: Mantrische Sprüche. Seelenübungen Band II (GA 268). Rudolf Steiner Verlag, Dornach 1999, p. 34, Draft, Notebook 1908.
137 Schiller, F.: Über die ästhetische Erziehung des Menschen in einer Reihe von Briefen, 1793 bis 1794.
138 Pütz, R. M.: Farbmeditation – Untersuchung von potenzierten Verfahren meditativer Malabläufe mit Pflanzenfarben als Basiserarbeitung für maltherapeutische Maßnahmen. Bertelsmann Verlag, Bielefeld 1991.
139 Steiner, R.: Meditative Betrachtungen und Anleitungen zur Vertiefung der Heilkunst (GA 316). Rudolf Steiner Verlag, Dornach 2008, p. 138.
140 Steiner, R.: Eurythmie als sichtbarer Gesang (GA 278). Rudolf Steiner Verlag, Dornach 2001, p. 49, Third lecture, Dornach, 21 February 1924.
141 Steiner, R.: Wie erlangt man Erkenntnisse der höheren Welten? (GA 10). Rudolf Steiner Verlag, Dornach 1992, p. 43 ff.
142 Ibid. p. 60 ff.
143 Anyone who would object that in a more detailed examination with a microscope the imitation could be distinguished from the real seed only shows that they have not understood what is important here. This is not about the precise manifestation to the sense of what we have in front of us, but that we use it to develop soul and spiritual forces.
144 From: Steiner, R.; Maryon, E.: Briefwechsel – Briefe – Sprüche – Skizzen 1912–1924 (GA 263/1). Rudolf Steiner Verlag, Dornach 1990.
145 Steiner, R.: Wahrspruchworte (GA 40). Rudolf Steiner Nachlassverwaltung, Dornach 1981, p. 140. Given for the art of eurythmy, Stuttgart, Christmas 1919.
146 Steiner, R.: Mantrische Sprüche. Seelenübungen Band II (GA 268). Rudolf Steiner Verlag, Dornach 1999, p. 296 ff. To Helene von Grunelius for the physicians, autumn 1923.
147 Steiner, R.: Meditative Betrachtungen und Anleitungen zur Vertiefung der Heilkunst (GA 316). Rudolf Steiner Verlag, Dornach 2008, p. 138, Eighth lecture, 9 January 1924.

148 Steiner, R.: Mantrische Sprüche. Seelenübungen Band II (GA 268). Rudolf Steiner Verlag, Dornach 1999, p. 97.
149 Steiner, R.: Eurythmie als sichtbare Sprache (GA 279), p. 238, Fourteenth lecture, Dornach, 11 July 1924.
150 Steiner, R.: Mantrische Sprüche. Seelenübungen Band II (GA 268). Rudolf Steiner Verlag, Dornach 1999, p. 195.
151 Ibid.
152 Ibid. p. 179.
153 Steiner, R.: Wahrspruchworte (GA 40), Rudolf Steiner Nachlassverwaltung, Dornach 1981, p. 116f., Lecture of 24 September 1919, for Helene Röchlin.
154 Steiner, R.: Das Zusammenwirken von Ärzten und Seelsorgern. Pastoral-Medizinischer Kurs (GA 318). Rudolf Steiner Verlag, Dornach 1994, p. 163.
155 Steiner, R.: Wahrspruchworte (GA 40). Rudolf Steiner Verlag, Dornach 1981, p. 116f.
156 Steiner, R.: Geisteswissenschaft und soziale Frage. In: Lucifer – Gnosis (GA 34). Rudolf Steiner Verlag, Dornach 1987.
157 Steiner, R.: Mantrische Sprüche. Seelenübungen Band II (GA 268). Rudolf Steiner Verlag, Dornach 1999, p. 309.
158 Steiner, R.: Mysteriengestaltungen (GA 232). Rudolf Steiner Verlag, Dornach 1987.
159 Steiner, R.: Das Osterfest als ein Stück Mysteriengeschichte der Menschheit (GA 233 a). Rudolf Steiner Verlag, Dornach 1991.
160 Steiner, R.: Landwirtschaftlicher Kurs (GA 327). Rudolf Steiner Verlag, Dornach 1999.
161 Steiner, R.: Das Zusammenwirken von Ärzten und Seelsorgern. Pastoral-Medizinischer Kurs (GA 318). Rudolf Steiner Verlag, Dornach 1994.
162 Steiner, R.: Mantrische Sprüche. Seelenübungen Band II (GA 268). Rudolf Steiner Verlag, Dornach 1999, p. 296.
163 Ibid. p. 299.
164 Ibid. p. 303.
165 Steiner, R.: Mysterienstätten des Mittelalters. Rosenkreuzertum und modernes Einweihungsprinzip (GA 233 a). Rudolf Steiner Verlag, Dornach 1991, p. 71.
166 Steiner, R.: Mantrische Sprüche. Seelenübungen Band II (GA 268). Rudolf Steiner Verlag, Dornach 1999, p. 303.
167 Cf. also Steiner, R.: Die Geheimwissenschaft im Umriss (GA 13). Rudolf Steiner Verlag, Dornach 1989.
168 Steiner, R.: Meditative Betrachtungen und Anleitungen zur Vertiefung der Heilkunst (GA 316). Rudolf Steiner Verlag, Dornach 2008.
169 Ibid. p. 177.

170 Steiner, R.: Mantrische Sprüche. Seelenübungen Band II (GA 268). Rudolf Steiner Verlag, Dornach 1999, p. 305.
171 Steiner, R.: Meditative Betrachtungen und Anleitungen zur Vertiefung der Heilkunst (GA 316). Rudolf Steiner Verlag, Dornach 2008, p. 208 ff.
172 Steiner, R.: Mantrische Sprüche. Seelenübungen Band II (GA 268). Rudolf Steiner Verlag, Dornach 1999, p. 306.
173 Steiner, R.: Meditative Betrachtungen und Anleitungen zur Vertiefung der Heilkunst (GA 316). Rudolf Steiner Verlag, Dornach 2008, p. 217.
174 Steiner, R.: Mantrische Sprüche. Seelenübungen Band II (GA 268). Rudolf Steiner Verlag, Dornach 1999, p. 317.
175 Ibid. p. 304.
176 Steiner, R.: Heilpädagogischer Kurs (GA 317). Rudolf Steiner Verlag, Dornach 1995, p. 154.
177 Ibid. p. 153.

Christof Wiechert

The Waldorf School

An Introduction

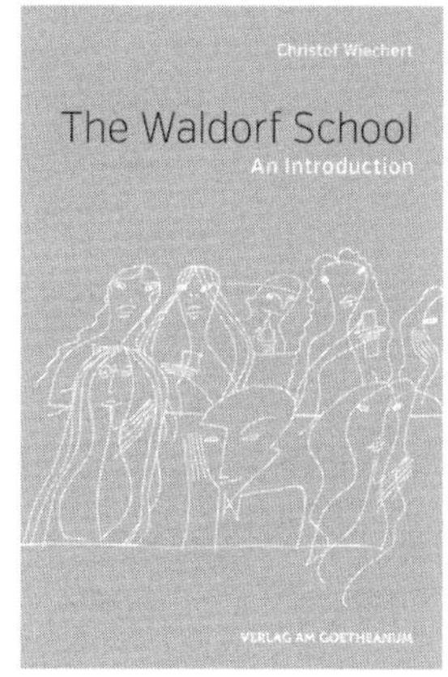

What is distinctive about Waldorf or Rudolf Steiner schools? How do their pedagogical aims relate to the wide range of educational provision available today? Many people have heard of these schools, but few know much about them.

Waldorf schools pursue an innovative educational practice that could enliven, inspire and renew many aspects of today's education system. This accessible and straightforward book describes the core concerns of Waldorf education and the current challenges it faces. It is intended for parents, teachers and trainee teachers, and anyone else who is interested in understanding what these schools are about, but who may not wish to grapple with some of the educational theories underlying this approach.

120 p., paperback, ISBN 978-3-7235-1539-6

Verlag am Goetheanum